Advance praise for *Grace*

"In her book, *Grace: A Child's Intimate Journey Through Ca[...]* Marchiano offers an honest and inspiring portrayal of her cancer experience through the eyes of a teenager and proves there is medicinal value in love and laughter. Melinda and I share a common bond. We are survivors. And we believe in the importance of empowering fellow survivors to live life on their own terms. By sharing her story, Melinda is giving a voice to this global epidemic that needs immediate attention. I am grateful to Melinda for having the courage to speak up and for her generosity in helping others fighting cancer."

—Lance Armstrong
Founder of the Lance Armstrong Foundation, seven-time Tour de France winner, and cancer survivor

"I have often said God gives children with cancer something extra. They are remarkable and inspiring people to be around. Melinda tells her story with such honesty and openness that you can't help but be touched and encouraged. This is sure to be a blessing to all who read it!"

—Jeff Foxworthy
Comedian, best-selling author, spokesperson for CURE Childhood Cancer Association, and honorary fundraising chairman for the Duke University Children's Hospital

"What Melinda has learned in fifteen years is far more than most people learn in a lifetime. Her attitude, faith, insights, and humor are a true inspiration."

—Ray Romano

"*Grace* is more than a book. It is a rare gem. With breathtaking insights and exquisite writing, as I read *Grace*, I kept wondering if Melinda was actually an award-winning author with multiple novels to her credit. No, in fact she is a 15-year-old cancer patient telling it like it is and she's utterly compelling."

—Kairol Rosenthal
Author of *Everything Changes: The Insider's Guide to Cancer in Your 20s and 30s*

"*Grace: A Child's Intimate Journey Through Cancer and Recovery* is a vivid and engaging description of a brave and articulate youth's encounter with cancer."

—Dr. Lee Hartwell
2001 Nobel Laureate, President & Director, Fred Hutchinson Cancer Research Center

"*Grace: A Child's Intimate Journey Through Cancer and Recovery* is required reading for anyone touched by cancer—parents, children, friends, and caregivers. It tells the story of a courageous girl through the perspective that is rarely heard—hers!

—Dr. Thomas J. Lynch
Director, Yale Cancer Center, Physician-in-Chief, Smilow Cancer Hospital

"Many people have written about their individual battles with cancer, some very beautifully. Melinda Marchiano tells the story of her cancer in a particularly engaging manner. Her message—that you are not alone and that you can prevail—will lift the spirits of many, particularly younger patients like her."

—Dr. Edward J. Benz
President, Dana-Farber Cancer Institute
Richard and Susan Smith Professor of Medicine
Professor of Pediatrics, Professor of Pathology
Harvard Medical School

"*Grace: A Child's Intimate Journey Through Cancer and Recovery* is a rare book—brave, inspiring, and empowering. Buy this book for a person with cancer, but read it first yourself. This uplifting story from 15-year-old Melinda will make your heart soar."

—Regina Ellis
Chief Executive Officer
Founder, Children's Cancer Association, www.JoyRx.org

"*Grace* is a remarkable book. Melinda tells every detail of her walk with cancer. Reading her words opened my eyes to the feelings that my 23-month-old daughter must have had but could not express: Alexa lost her battle to Neuroblastoma in 2004. We realized that Alexa's trials were to give rise to a greater purpose, and now her light shines through our Foundation, just as Melinda's shines through her written word."

—Joann M. Nawrocki
Alexa Nawrocki Pediatric Cancer Foundation, Inc.

"Clearly Melinda is articulate, open and courageous beyond her years. As a teenager, and even as an adult, I can easily fall into a 'why me, it's not fair' mentality over the most trivial thing. It's easy to overlook so much on a daily basis, and Melinda's book is a reminder to be grateful no matter what our situation is. She is truly inspiring. I believe that her book will be a gift to many people, young and old . . . the survivors and the families."

—Yvonne Jung
Actress, *Criminal Minds, Third Watch, The Sopranos*

"There is great comfort in knowing that another young person has faced cancer and has overcome its many challenges. Melinda's personal story lights that difficult path and offers encouragement and hope to the patient, siblings, and parents."

—Moody D. Wharam, Jr., MD, FACR, FASTRO
Professor of Radiation Oncology
Department of Radiation Oncology and Molecular Radiation Sciences
The Sidney Kimmel Comprehensive Cancer Center at Johns Hopkins

"Upon seeing Melinda at first, her eyes told that she was an old soul. When listening, her lips spoke with much wisdom, and now when reading her book this same passion for life is shared in her words as she experiences weakness and triumph in life. Melinda is of great influence and *Grace* lifts up the reader to show anyone can conquer with will power and . . . well . . . Grace."

—Matt Hackney
Chief Executive Officer
TheSBON, HardMagic, MOVFitness
Author of *The Summit of Success*, *The Fire Within*, and *Published!*

"Thank you so much for bringing this to my attention. Good for you, your strength will be a light house for others. I'd love to endorse your book. Having lost family members to cancer, I think your book will be an inspiration for others in time of great need. You have an undeniable open channel of talent and a voice that needs to be heard! Much love and success."

—Anthony Ruivivar
Actor, "Third Watch" "Tropic Thunder" "CSI"

"Melinda's sharing of her courageous battle with pediatric cancer is truly inspiring. Hopefully other young adults who are dealing with this disease will read her story and find companionship and strength in their journeys as well. Melinda exemplifies *Grace* to the fullest degree."

—Kathleen A. Casey
Founder and President, Bear Necessities Pediatric Cancer Foundation

"Melinda tells her story of personal challenge and growth with openness and style. Her inspiring message of perseverance, healing, and God's grace will inspire all who read this beautiful book."

—R. Diane Schlesinger, M.D.
Adult, Adolescent, and Child Psychiatry

"Thank you so much for forwarding a sample of your wonderful, inspiring book. Your courage and talent shine through your words and insights into your challenges and struggles. My best wishes on your success"

—Barton J. Blinder, M.D.
Faculty: Clinical Professor, Dept. Psychiatry and Human Behavior, School of Medicine University of California, Irvine

GRACE

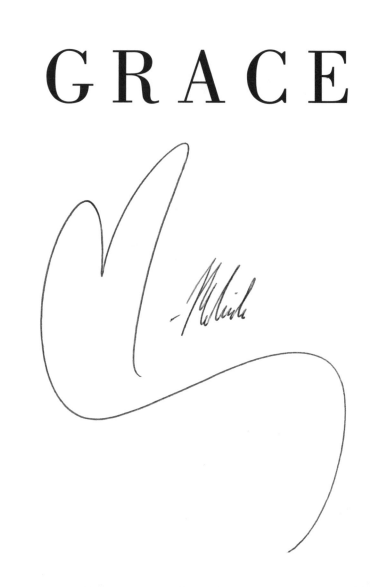

a memoir

GRACE

a child's intimate journey
through cancer and recovery

melinda marchiano

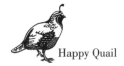

Happy Quail

Published by Happy Quail
San Luis Obispo, CA
www.happyquail.net

Distributed by Greenleaf Book Group LLC

For ordering information or special discounts for bulk purchases, please contact Greenleaf Book Group LLC at PO Box 91869, Austin, TX 78709, 512.891.6100.

Design and composition by Greenleaf Book Group LLC and Bumpy Design

Cover design by Greenleaf Book Group LLC
Photography by D. Lee Marchiano, except where noted

Unless otherwise noted, scripture taken from the NEW AMERICAN STANDARD BIBLE, Copyright ©1960, 1962, 1963, 1968, 1971, 1972, 1973, 1975, 1977, 1995 by the Lockman Foundation. Used with permission.

"The Waiting" lyrics by Tom Petty. Printed with permission of Wixen Music Publishing.

Publisher's Cataloging-In-Publication Data
(Prepared by The Donohue Group, Inc.)

Marchiano, Melinda.
  Grace : a memoir : a child's intimate journey through cancer and recovery / Melinda Marchiano ; photography by D. Lee Marchiano. -- 2nd ed.

    p. : ill. ; cm.

  ISBN: 978-0-9842712-0-7

  1. Marchiano, Melinda. 2. Cancer in children--Patients--Biography. I. Marchiano, D. Lee. II. Title.

RC281.C4 M27 2010
618.92/994/092   2010927904

Part of the Tree Neutral™ program, which offsets the number of trees consumed in the production and printing of this book by taking proactive steps, such as planting trees in direct proportion to the number of trees used: www.treeneutral.com

TreeNeutral™

Printed in the United States of America on acid-free paper

10 11 12 13 14 15   10 9 8 7 6 5 4 3 2 1

Second Edition

ACKNOWLEDGMENTS

This book is for:

My loving family:
Mom, Dad, Nicholas, Dean, and Larry

My loving extended family:
Gramma, Poppy, Uncle Jeff, Aunt Sharon, Uncle Greg, Aunt Valerie, G-Pop, Grandma M., Uncle Bruce, "the cousins," Aunt Ruth and Uncle Wen, Sissy, Aunt Marion, Aunt Phyllis and Lou, Aunt Barbara, Lory and Jim, Uncle Abbott and Aunt Muriel, the Johnson families, AJ, and the Mitchellinos

My incredible medical team:
Dr. Dan Greenfield, Nurse Pam, Jaynie, Robyn, Nanci, Zippy, Dr. Howarth, Dr. Gonzalez, Nurses: Cyndi, Gail, Sue, Lisa, Paralee, Kristy, Amalia, Debra, Sioban, Novice, Nancy, Jen, and Isabell; Dr. Keshen, Dr. Kelts, Dr. Willsey, Dr. Pickert, Dr. Josh, Dr. Weisenburger, Kym, Sylvia, Ed, Louis, Don, Sandra, Dr. A., Carlos, Heidi, and Cottage Hospital therapy dogs: Sammy, Scruffy, Sugar, Dottie, Echo, Paloma, Carmel, Ralph, Ryder, and especially Rowan

Others at Cottage Hospital/The Children's Miracle Network/Surprises:
Arnie for his songs, Audrie Krause, Maria Zate, Jeff Martin, Paula Lopez, Alan Rose, Rusty, Jorge, Glenn, Collette Briere, Joe, Rachel, Jake and Aliyah, Patricia Barker, Tom Kenny, Paula Deen, and Lance Armstrong

Amazing friends:

JY, Vicki, and Schyler, the Valdez family, Johanna, Gregg and Karen Kaufman, Casey Roberts, Debi, Suze, Lynn, the Alessi family, Tim Stipanuk, Karl, Lydia, Mary Ann, Jeff Ketcham, Ausma, Diana, Dick and Patty Melsheimer, Carolyn Abernathy, Matt Hackney, Ralph and Carolyn Miner, Ric, Maricella, Lou, Gene and Bev Kai, the Fischers, the Kozlowskis, the Boyds, the loving ladies from PEO, Marty and Mary, the Krzystons, Mary White, the Chavarria family, my school friends: Mr. Houchin, Barbara Miller, Ms. Lopez, Mr. Gracia, Ms. Jenssen, Ms. Belo, Mr. Ritchie, Mr. and Mrs. Long, Mr. Hubbell, Mrs. Petrusky, Ms. Brooks; my church friends: Arroyo Grande United Methodist Church, Gloria Dei Church in Orcutt, and Clearview United Methodist Church in St. Petersburg, Florida; my post office friends: Debbie, Barbara, and Connie; my Vons friends: Susan, Donna, and Jake; my Jamba Juice friends, Zac and Jamie; the Teddy Bear Cancer Foundation, Mr. Travis Wilson, the Teddy Bear Man, Devon and Sammie, the Tony Stewart Foundation, Stefanie at Make-A-Wish Foundation, my dance teachers: Ms. Shelagh, Ms. Cynthia, Michelle, Jackie, Elena, Dana, and Drew; and my fellow dancers at the Academy of Dance in San Luis Obispo.

FOREWORD

WHEN I FIRST MET MELINDA, she was about to complete her final week of chemotherapy for Hodgkin lymphoma. Neither one of us knew at the time that she was only halfway through the journey on which cancer would bring her. Now, like most people who meet Melinda, I knew instantly that this was a young woman who possessed special qualities. After only a few minutes with Melinda, it became clear to me that she has a way of interacting with the world and the people in it that maximizes joy, meaning, and above all else, laughter. Melinda's sense of humor is fantastic, sarcastic, nonstop, and even perhaps a bit wicked. It's difficult to be around Melinda and not find yourself smiling at her jokes and realizing that yes, it's okay to laugh at bad situations. Although I only interacted with her during that last week of chemotherapy, subsequent emails, photographs, and now this wonderful book you hold in front of you all confirm my initial impressions of Melinda: this is a girl worth knowing and learning from.

In this, her first book, aptly named *Grace,* Melinda takes us on the many-year journey that is cancer. In fact, by the time you reach the end of her story, you realize that Melinda's adventures are truly just beginning. Her clear and clever articulation of the struggles inherent to cancer impressed me greatly. She teaches the reader at every point along the way, and she is not afraid to share with you the brutal truth about being a teenager with cancer. This includes the emotional struggles of being treated for a life-threatening, and certainly life-changing, illness.

However, this book is far from being a depressing novel about the trials and tribulations of cancer, and in fact, Melinda's memoir is quite the opposite. It is a surprisingly uplifting tale and a celebration of how the human spirit can prevail over the challenges life throws our way. It is the story of how with the right attitude and loving support, those struggles can be overcome and lead to greatness. Oftentimes while reading Melinda's story, I had to pause to remember that this was being written by a young teenager and simply shake my head in amazement at the way she so elegantly expresses the nuances of battling cancer. Most importantly, Melinda shares with the reader that the major challenge of confronting cancer is more than dealing with the physical symptoms. It is coming to terms with the way that cancer changes one's perspective about what it means to be alive and how the experience can transform your very own identity.

Grace is a book that speaks to me personally on many levels. It is an absolute page-turner, bursting with genuine insights about the field of caring for children with cancer. As a pediatric oncologist, my professional life is immersed daily in the world of childhood cancer, and Melinda does an impressive job of describing both the good and the bad that can be found in this land of sick children. I also had Hodgkin lymphoma as a teenager and could relate personally to what Melinda describes. Many times while reading *Grace* I would find myself nodding my head and saying aloud, "That's it! She hit the nail on the head." Melinda's approach is direct and forceful. She's not afraid to tell it like it is. I believe Melinda's book has the potential to shape the national discussion on the effects of cancer in children and young adults.

One of the powers of *Grace* is its ability to take you safely through the world of missed diagnoses, painful procedures, awful complications, and lingering late effects. Just when you feel like you can stand no more and that your heart is full of sorrow, Melinda lets you know that it's okay to feel bad and even joke about it too. After reading several passages, you will find yourself laughing aloud at Melinda's terrific sense of humor and her sarcastic wit—and laughing in situations where you would normally expect to be crying! It is this fresh perspective that allows you to be carried through Melinda's journey at top speed, turning page after page to see how it will end and how Melinda will cope with the next round of nausea or undiagnosed treatment-related problems.

Throughout the joking and even the tears, Melinda continues to teach the reader the importance of the support of family and friends through the cancer experience. It is not Melinda alone who overcomes the struggles in her life, but the loving-kindness of nurses, janitors, professional ballerinas, and even strangers at the gas station or in the supermarket. Although cancer can be scary, Melinda teaches us why you don't need to go through it alone and, in fact, how supporting those with cancer can be rewarding both for you and for the patient. By the end of *Grace,* the reader has perhaps one of the best recipes I have ever read for "when life gives you lemons, make them into lemonade." Be forewarned, this lemonade may come shooting out your nose in laughter as you read the pages of Melinda's story!

Joshua Schiffman, MD
Assistant Professor
Pediatric Hematology/Oncology
University of Utah

GRACE

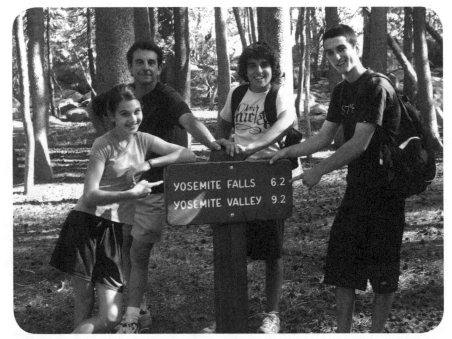

Dad, Dean, Nicholas, and I after our family hike to the top of Yosemite Falls, June 2007.

ONE

IT WAS JUNE 2007, and my family and I were on vacation in beautiful Yosemite National Park. We had just set out for the day, our destination—the top of Yosemite Falls. The twelve-and-a-half-mile hike started in a small campground and wound through gorgeous forests, flowering meadows, and massive rock formations before reaching the top of the famous falls. My mom, dad, two brothers, and I were all excited and ready for adventure. As we started off on the long hike, I began to realize how weak I felt. How could I feel so tired? I danced multiple days a week and was in great physical shape. I became slightly frustrated as my dad and I brought up the rear. Normally, I would be skipping out in front, not shoved to the back by a simple hill climb.

I vividly remember the top of the falls. It was the closest thing to heaven that my human mind could conjure up. We stood on a giant stone that, at one point, suddenly cut off and plunged miles and miles into the valley below. It was as if we gazed upon the entire world from that one single point. But as my eyes gobbled up the incredible view, I noticed that I was dizzy; my head felt weird. I felt . . . unwell. I was thirteen, at the prime of my youth. It didn't make sense. Little did I know, as I sat atop the world, what the next two years would bring and how fast that innocent, little girl I knew would have to grow up.

Fast-forwarding to August . . . my mom and I were in the backseat of my grandparents' Buick and on our way to Crescent City, in Northern California, to see my Uncle Jeff and to celebrate my Aunt Sharon's birthday. At this checkpoint in my steadily declining health, I was feeling ill all the time. However, my physical symptoms weren't corresponding with any particular sickness. Having had multiple bad colds that year, I blamed any discomfort on that.

But there was a deeper, eerie feeling of a general lack of well-being. It was a feeling that permeated my entire body, and I felt a sensation of it disconnecting and slipping away from me. It still gives me the chills to this day. I felt as if my body didn't belong to me any longer, that it was a slave to some dark force that controlled its fate. I blamed my mind for that horrible sense and was actually a little concerned that I was mentally ill—going crazy. All of these thoughts rolled around in my head as we took on the winding, nauseating, mountain roads. I was dizzy, queasy, and then I began to feel the slightest, not pain, but a . . . something in my chest. I found it difficult to take a deep breath, and I tried to calm down and relax. I couldn't get sick *here*; where would we go?

As the trip went on, I felt worse and worse. At my uncle's house, I remember going to sleep at night, lying on my back. It felt like I had someone sitting on my chest, or forcefully pushing down on my heart and lungs. I could barely get in a normal breath. Dizzy and light-headed, I was becoming frightened. Was I having a heart attack or something? Then I turned on my side. Hmm . . . I could breathe easier, and I could finally fall asleep.

In the following month or so, my mom watched me closely. If I felt any worse, we were going to go to the doctor to get a blood test. I admit that, at the time, I had never gotten a blood test, and I was absolutely terrified of the idea. For that reason, I probably made myself think I was feeling better, even though it was blatantly obvious to me that I was becoming sicker. It became a daily battle, and I began to realize just how horrible I felt. However, I was frightened and didn't want to freak out anybody else. That would scare me even more. But I knew inside that something was very wrong. I couldn't take it anymore. We made an appointment. And so, the age of Dr. A. and the many wrong diagnoses began.

⌒

I curled up on the floor in our living room, my eyes two leaky faucets. Our dog, Larry, looked worried and shook as I broke down. The following day was my first blood test, and I was mortified. But even more so, the emotional and physical exhaustion of being ill day after day was setting in. Luckily, I was home-schooled, but each day I pushed myself to go to dance, take Larry on a walk, and do other simple daily activities. I was constantly cold, my lips were blue, my face as white as a sheet. There was no hiding the obvious. I had to get help. And at that moment of utter helplessness and trauma, I began to peel back the layers of who I truly was, and we began to drill to the core of my suffering. The problem? It was hidden deeply within me, and rock solid.

Tweety Bird smiled at me from the Band-Aid carefully placed on the table next to me. I stared at his cute, beaky grin and squeezed my mom's hand as hard as I could; tears rolled down my face. And then, as quickly as it began, my first blood test was over. I got out of there as swiftly as I could, and I clearly recall eating a mountain of French toast once I returned home and my fast was over.

Sitting at the kitchen table, I was unable to focus on my math lesson. My mind wandered, my arm hurt, and my heart sat heavily within me. Looking back, this day is a slice of heaven compared to what I would have to endure. I have no doubt that God prepared me for everything I had to go through. And now, with almost 125 pokes behind me, a tiny stick of the needle is like brushing my teeth—something I just have to do.

"She's anemic!" Dr. A. shouted in her gruff voice.

My blood tests revealed that my iron count was low, which is sometimes common for teenage girls. Mom and I sighed in relief as Dr. A. wrote a prescription for an iron supplement. We were thrilled that my illness was "easy to fix," and we immediately screeched to a halt in front of Vons supermarket, to load up on spinach and red meat. We picked up the iron supplement as soon as we could, and I began to take it, with full belief that the vile, horrible-tasting liquid would magically cure me.

I could not swallow pills, and the most intense medication I had ever taken was that pink, cherry-flavored Tylenol. I gulped and chugged down my medication as fast as I could without gagging. The mega-pack of bendy straws in our cupboard helped prevent my teeth from getting stained; however, as a result of the memory of the horrid taste, I have now refrained from using straws. Within a week, Mom noticed that I was sinking lower and even lower into my chair, and my sheet-white face began to resemble a ghost. It was not good . . . we had to keep looking.

I smeared on some of my new cinnamon lip gloss as we, once again, headed out the door for Dr. A.'s. That lip gloss is now in the trash, still half full. Why must good things be ruined by bad memories? At this time, I started getting blood tests almost every week. It got so ridiculous that Carlos, the man from the lab, had to tell me to come back because my veins had too many scars to draw blood. I continued to get wrongly diagnosed.

I still remember the deep, gut laugh that escaped my mom when Dr. A. announced, "She's depressed!"

Even I had to chuckle at that one . . . there was just no way. Mom diligently kept pushing for more tests. Each time, Dr. A. looked at us like we were nuts, but she got out her pad and pen and, reluctantly, obliged our requests. I am still very thankful that she listened to us, despite her doubt.

In the following weeks, I received an echocardiogram, more blood tests, and a kidney ultrasound. Besides a slight murmur, my heart was fine, and the ultrasound also showed no abnormal signs. To be perfectly honest, I was becoming flustered that we weren't finding anything. I hoped and prayed that we would soon discover the culprit and that, whatever the heck it was, there would be an easy solution. I would lie in bed at night and cry. It seemed like every night, I would pour my heart out to my mom, who sat on my bed and held my hand.

In the midst of my misery, I heard her calm, reassuring voice, "We are going to keep searching until we find out what it is," Mom whispered.

Wanting to believe her, and making myself believe her, deep in my soul, I'm not quite sure that I did.

Thank God for the Internet. I know that it can be slow at times, and it can be aggravating, but seriously, it's pretty amazing. Mom spent hours upon hours looking over my tests, meticulously searching for what each result meant. She found out that the SED rate of my blood was higher than normal, which can be a signal of inflammation in the body. She was determined to discover if inflammation was, in fact, the cause of my anemia. If our search proved unsuccessful, the next step was to see a rheumatologist in Fresno.

Also at this time, I began to suffer extremely emotionally. No one believed I was sick, and they claimed, "You look fine."

It was wishful thinking. I was told that I needed to eat burgers and drink shakes to feel better, and I grew very angry that few trusted me. I was in my body and they were not; it was as simple as that. However, my mom remained my support, and she and I continued to get closer as our deep understanding of each other grew. Our spirits and souls began to intertwine, like two ivy branches wrapping and twisting around each other . . . becoming one.

I sighed and gave Mom one of my very convincing "I'm okay" smiles. I sat in yet another doctor's office, the paper on the table crunching underneath me. On the wall hung a bulletin board, with dozens of pictures of their patients. Their innocent eyes pierced my heart, and I, at last, noticed they were all bald. I had only noticed their little, glowing smiles and twinkling eyes, but I then began to see details. IV pumps were at their sides, nurses posed with them, and a few had "In Memory" delicately printed in the corner. The room also had inspirational quotes hung in various places along the freshly painted walls. One, that grew to become my favorite, instantly stood out and captured my attention.

"We are, each of us angels with only one wing; and we can only fly by embracing one another." —Luciano de Crescenzo

That quote reached right in and grabbed my soul. As I gazed at it, the large door swung open, and a woman walked in. Dr. Howarth is an oncologist/hematologist who Mom looked up on the Internet. It was a "see who takes our insurance" deal. I had gotten up fairly early, dragged my exhausted butt into the car, and Mom and I made the hour-and-a-half drive to Santa Barbara. This was the very first time I laid eyes on Cottage Hospital, a place I would soon know all too well.

My focus shifted to Dr. Howarth as she smiled and stated, "Hello," in her soft, British accent.

My plaster smile emerged, and I greeted her back. She assumed her position atop her wheely stool—it looked fun. I wanted a ride. She then gently asked me to describe the symptoms I was having. I became very hot, almost nervous. A lump formed in my throat as I struggled to find the right words to interpret how I felt. My eyes became glassy with tears, and I explained, as clearly as I could, the daily battle with being ill. With each word, my language became more indistinguishable. I didn't want to be there, and I desired so greatly to return to my spot on the couch, where my body fit perfectly within the indent I had formed in the cushion.

How do you tell someone you don't feel well? Dr. Howarth drilled me with questions, but none received a straight answer. I couldn't confirm anything, and I became frustrated and at a loss for words. No earthly verbal communication could possibly suffice to share the eerie, disturbing presence I felt within me.

Dr. Howarth left the room, and I changed into the latest, hottest, hospital fashion—not. It was the popular diamond pattern, the diamond pattern that, come December, would get thrown up on by yours truly. Speaking of puking, I recall some major nausea occurring as Dr. Howarth performed a thorough, and I mean *thorough*, examination of me. I'm not sure if my queasiness stemmed from something I ate or from complete loss of all dignity. Once I was back in my own clothes, walking out the door, I finally began to relax. Dr. Howarth ordered yet another request for the lab vampires to suck out my blood. She pointed to the children on the bulletin board.

"Don't worry," she reassured, "you're not one of them."

I picked up a few pieces of Halloween candy from the front desk and began down the hall. Just then, I saw a man burst out of a doorway, dancing and beaming from ear to ear. A young girl in pajamas smiled and giggled in her wheelchair. The two exchanged high fives as they celebrated the girl's blood counts. This was Dr. Dan, and he was doing his famous "happy dance," although we did not know it at the time. I watched the way he was with the girl as we strolled by, seeing them laugh and play joyfully.

Once they disappeared around the corner and out of view, I thought, "Wow, what a cool guy."

It is ironic that he should be the one to accompany me during some of my darkest hours.

The days wore on. It was now November, and the holidays and *The Nutcracker* were fast approaching. I had been attending all of my dance rehearsals, struggling through the long Saturdays before coming home to collapse on the couch. I remember one beautiful, clear, warm Saturday when I decided to sit outside after rehearsal. Plunking my bottom down in the sunshine, I looked around at the blue sky, lush grass, and the big Sequoia tree in our front yard. It all seemed different. The colors weren't as bright, and I didn't get that pure, peaceful feeling I normally got. In fact, it was like I was watching the world through a camera that couldn't focus. Everything was a faint blur. Trying hard to clear my foggy vision, I blinked my eyes wildly, but all remained the same. I returned to the house, devastated that I could not even enjoy God's gorgeous day.

I kept on dancing and dancing, doing the only thing, I believe, that kept me sane during that time. But during class, though, I was terribly weak, and I became aware of a little thing I like to call The Dolphin Cough. It was a blessing from hell. Coughing incessantly, I barked the same high-pitched squeals of a dolphin. The girls in my class would chuckle, and I would too. I would play with them by flapping my arms like flippers. It became an ongoing joke. But they didn't see me at home, curled up in a ball on the couch, hacking my brains out until I nearly passed out. I can still see the high-eyebrow look that Dr. A. gave my mom and me, as I described my unique cough at my next visit.

I imagined her thinking, "Wow, girl, you have major problems."

Apparently, my problems were beyond her knowledge, because she handed us a referral to a local pediatrician. But I can't complain. She, once again, whipped out her pad of paper and prescribed me some medicine. She also ordered one of the most crucial tests that contributed to my diagnosis. It was the chest X-ray that my mom requested. Taking some major convincing on our part, Dr. A. finally succumbed. Mom stood her ground until we got what we wanted.

I thank God I have a mom who is so driven and strong willed. Without her, I know wholeheartedly, I would not be here. Initially, we just wanted to be sure that my lungs were functioning properly and that there were no visible respiratory problems. We did not have a clue that what we would find would shock us all.

I wish that my mind could be permanently wiped clean of the memories of my cough medicine. I want so much to be able to see that little, evil, orange bottle in the cabinet and not involuntarily shiver and cringe. Imagine the most rancid, disgusting substance on planet Earth and multiply it by a thousand. Wah-lah! Behold—my cough medicine. I can recall myself scrunched up in a roly-poly position while I desperately downed Halls and warm tea . . . nothing worked.

Then the day came . . . the day our eyes were opened to just how serious this all was. The day of my chest X-ray, Mom and I sat in very uncomfortable chairs as we waited for my name to be called. Trying to enjoy the outdated magazines, my mind couldn't focus on anything. Britney Spears, or someone, stared at me until I heard my name. I went in, took off all I had on (which was getting old), and put on one of those stylish, XXXXL hospital gowns. Some dude squished me up against a target. I held my breath, and snap—I was out of there and on my way to dance.

A few days later, we got the results. We were onto something. My chest X-ray showed a slight abnormality, which I didn't think much of at the time. Having had a cyst removed from my chest as a newborn, there was a possibility that it might just be leftover scar tissue. Whatever it was, we all agreed that we had best schedule a CT scan to further investigate.

At this time, we met Dr. Irma Gonzalez. This sweet, caring woman will always have a special place deep in my heart. Hearing her calm voice, and seeing her warm smile, I immediately trusted and respected her. My first visit with Dr. Gonzalez was the same old "strip and get into the gown" routine. I received another blood test and also did the glorious pee-in-the-cup test. My CT scan was scheduled for the next day. We were on a medical roll . . . unfortunately.

Crap, that following day is just too clear in my mind. It was a Tuesday afternoon, and we pulled into the parking lot at Digital Medical Imaging. I was feeling tense and nervous because I knew I would have to have an IV put in. It was my first of so many IVs that I've lost count. Also, I was kind of crabby because I didn't do well with the whole fasting thing. We ran into a friend, John Gutshall, and we laughed and joked with him a bit. I pretend laughed. I recall looking down at my leg; it tapped impatiently.

Before I had the chance to get comfortable, they called me in. After changing, like Superman, I walked into a cold, dimly lit room. The doughnut-shaped machine hummed . . . deep and low. I told myself I could do it. But just before the technician inserted my IV, I began to cry. The woman mocked me, and I cried harder. Doing the death grip on Mom's hand, I braved the stick, and the worst part was over—at least what I thought was the worst part. Mom gave my hand one last squeeze as she exited and went into the control room. You know those moments, both good and bad, where life seems to stop for a second? Yep, I had one of those, lying alone in the CT scanner in that haunting room.

⌒

Mom shared the story of what happened in the other room, later on in my treatment. I know that we are supposed to forgive, but I admit that it took me a long time to forgive the technician for her cruelty. Mom described herself as extremely concerned that day and the worry obviously showed on her face. She had seen so many chilling photos on the Internet of CT results that were horribly wrong. She stared at the screen and, I imagine, held her breath.

The technician, sensing my mom's anxiety, blurted, "Oooooo, Mom looks scared."

When I heard this, I was so disgusted, I could not even speak. Her taunting, and complete lack of compassion, made me gag, and it still does. This day was one of the scariest days Mom and I have ever endured, and that woman did not have the right to make it worse. To top it off, suddenly a picture loaded on the computer screen in the control room. Mom says that every ounce of blood drained from her body. The picture was exactly like those she had seen on the Internet. It was awful, unreal.

Like any parent would do, Mom didn't tell me about what she saw. She didn't want to freak me out and, looking back, I'm glad that I didn't know. It gave me just a little more time to still be myself—to feel somewhat in control of my life.

⌒

"I think we finally found it," Mom prepared me as she shut off the car.

"I think that we might have found the culprit . . . I just have a feeling."

I stared at one old, worn-out paint line in the parking lot. It was white and rough, stopping at one point before continuing on. Strange, the things we remember. I could literally re-create the entire experience . . . not that I would want to or anything.

The last thing Mom told me, as I stumbled out of the car, was, "Whatever we find, we're going to get it."

Why are doctor's office clocks so loud? They seem to "death tick," each second a loud clunk that makes your heart leap. The room was icy cold, and I had goose bumps, accompanied by the chills. I examined the little, clear jar of cotton balls for a few minutes, and then I heard the door opening. Every hair on my body stood on end. I had a weird tickle in my stomach that I blamed on breakfast. Dr. Gonzalez wore her usual glowing grin, but a look in her eyes displayed great concern. She greeted us and perched atop her stool. All was quiet, for just a moment, and then she began.

"Well, we found something on your CT."

She hesitated, and a millisecond of relief came over me, but it was just that, one teeny tiny ounce of joy before my entire world melted around me. Dr. Gonzalez looked in our eyes and stated, as calmly as she could, my pitiful situation. A mass sat in my chest cavity, with major arteries running through it at all angles.

What?! I had never even heard of a chest cavity. How did it get there? Mom and I glanced at one another . . . I couldn't keep it together any longer. I broke down. Like a scared little puppy, I blubbered, the room blurring behind my curtain of tears. Immediately, in a flash, both Dr. Gonzalez and Mom were by my side, hugging me.

"I was up all night thinking about this. I really didn't want to have to tell you," she confessed.

Feeling numb, and like I was floating, I suddenly became aware of my chest. Just knowing that some alien thing was present, had invaded me, made my chest hurt. Shortness of breath overcame me. Something cheated me out of normal health, and I felt complete lack of control. What would happen now? Would I need surgery? If so, would my entire chest cavity have to be cut open, vital arteries severed, before piecing me back together? At first I feared surgery, but once determining it was nearly impossible, I became more fearful. It couldn't have been *my* body she was talking about. It just couldn't be. How *could* it be?

Dr. G. left the room, giving Mom and me some time alone. As the door clicked shut, I fell into her arms. I don't recall how long we remained there, wrapped tightly around one another, but eventually Dr. Gonzalez returned. She carried a small piece of paper in her hand. That paper held the name of Dr. Daniel Greenfield, the man who would become my hero and lifesaver.

I looked at the beautiful Nipomo hills as we drove up to our local Vons. We needed orange juice, I remember. Everything seemed different, appeared different, and emitted a grim feeling. Mom went in, but I remained in the car. I watched for her to disappear into the store, and then I collapsed into an ocean of tears.

"Lord, please give me strength," I pleaded.

It was pitiful and, luckily, no one saw me. Turning on my "windshield wipers," I gathered myself together. Taking the deepest breath I could, I told myself that I could do it—I would make it through.

That night was Parent Day at dance, and Mom set her digital camera on the center console of our truck. I was still in a somewhat mummified state, and a somber expression stayed glued on my face. Mom and I were both quiet . . . there was nothing to talk about, yet everything in the world to discuss. Our car sped along our main street, and beginning to forget about my pain, I noticed something else. The most incredible sunset lit up the sky, with reds, oranges, and every color in between. It seemed as if God lit the vast, blue horizon on fire, and the sight was truly overwhelming. How a view can be *that* magnificent, I have no idea. Its vibrant colors and unbelievable presence poured hope into my empty, deprived soul.

It was God saying, "*I am always with you.*"

Distraction dominated my conscience as my dance instructor taught us combinations. I tried my hardest to rid my mind of the fact that I was dancing with a giant mass, a terrible blob that limited both my breathing and blood flow. Making situations seem a lot better than they actually are was becoming one of my strongest assets. I looked to Mom, who sat in a black, paint-chipped chair. Our eyes connected, and I saw sheer terror within them.

Pointing to her, I mouthed, "Are you okay?"

She nodded. She was a tough one . . . still is. Mom then pointed back to me and mimed the same question. Also nodding, I tried to be strong for her. We both struggled individually, yet we fought to be each other's crutches. We could summon no power for ourselves, yet we somehow managed to muster up a speck for one another. So, occasionally, we would simultaneously give each other "the look" . . . both of us trying to reassure the other.

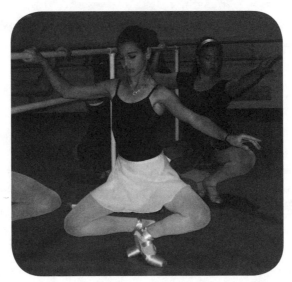

Parent Day at dance, 2007.

"Dancers are athletes of God." —Albert Einstein

TWO

"GOOD MORNING, young lady," he announced while shaking my hand. "And how are you today?"

This was Dr. Dan Greenfield, the gentle, comical, white-coatless doctor I would come to love. At the very first sight of him, he came off as more of a friend, with nothing other than a stethoscope perched atop his shoulders. I couldn't put my finger on it, but he took on the appearance of a cartoon character . . . one that creates warm, fuzzy feelings and makes you grin from ear to ear. He was Ernie . . . or Bert . . . or maybe Elmo? Well, whatever memorable Muppet he resembled, he had a tranquil, serene, yet strong presence that became very apparent the moment he walked in.

After examining me briefly, he listened intently to everything I had to say. This is a trait that I admire so much about Dr. Dan. He not only listens but also genuinely, wholeheartedly cares. Immediately, I respected his passionate knowledge, deep wisdom, and, especially, the true concern and understanding he portrayed. It overflowed from his heart, like a pond just after a newly fallen rain.

Suddenly, Dr. Dan opened the door. He asked me to go out into the hall, specifically, I remember, to draw a picture. Extremely confused, I went along with what he wished. My shoes squeaked as I waddled out the door. Hospital floors are funny like that, extra squeaky. Give me some wet shoes and turn me loose in there . . . I'll be entertained all day.

Anyway, I glanced up from the realistic picture of SpongeBob I had begun drawing and saw the large door shut tightly behind Dr. Dan. Oh, gotcha. He wanted to talk to Mom and Dad. Trying to guess what they were discussing, I formed two perfectly round circles for the eyes. I assumed it wasn't too good, stuff that I shouldn't hear or it would scare me. I'm not sure if I appreciated it at the time. I couldn't decide.

A cheerful nurse walked up to me as I spaced out, filling in each tiny gap with a yellow crayon. I don't recall exactly what she said, but Pam, who would become lovingly referred to as Nurse Pam, treated me as if I were her own.

"Don't worry," she comforted, "moms and dads are always concerned. They just love you."

I had almost finished coloring the ocean around SpongeBob as the door swung open once again. I'm not sure how long I slumped over at that little kiddy table. Time had become a nothing—virtually pointless, meaningless.

⌒

Mom and Dad's appearances had changed, I noticed, as I was called back to rejoin them. I hopped up onto the crunchy paper table, drawing in hand. As if each little feature weighed a ton, my parents' faces sunk with the weight of something, though I did not know what. The door closed. Click. Click. Dr. Dan dove into all sorts of information. The words alone were frightening but, for some reason, when they came out of his mouth, they did not take on the same persona. Making it all sound so simple, he even joked with me.

"You are going to get a PET scan tomorrow, and no, this is not a scan of your pet."

I chuckled, feeling very comfortable with him. He explained that he believed my symptoms were those of Valley Fever or Hodgkin lymphoma. A biopsy was mentioned, something that, I admit, was scary for me at the time. After asking what both illnesses' treatment would entail, I don't recall what he said about Valley Fever. Maybe it's because his answer for Hodgkin lymphoma was so profound, yet so simple.

"We melt it with medicine," he declared.

This was Dr. Dan's tender way of crudely stating, "You get chemo, kid."

Thanks Dr. Dan . . . fooled me.

"Even when we feel we can't be strong, we can still be a source
of strength for others." —Noah benShea

"Hi Cole," I greeted him as the cute little boy gazed up at me through his round glasses.

A few wisps of blonde hair atop his head made his blue-green eyes pop.

"I have something for you," I announced, walking into the play/waiting room.

He stared at me, and I continued.

"Nurse Pam told me you like SpongeBob too."

He nodded shyly.

"I drew this for you," I said quietly, my arm outstretched, presenting the drawing.

Cole was extremely shy, and he hid his face in the stroller. Taking the picture, his mom held it before him.

"Look Cole," she gasped with excitement.

Just then, his little head emerged from the corner of the stroller. He eyed the brightly colored SpongeBob and the note, "To Cole, from Melinda," neatly written at the bottom.

No smile came out. He just stared, but I could tell he liked it. Nurse Pam had told me all about Cole out in the hall, and it felt so good to do something for him.

"Thank you," his mom stated graciously.

Making for the door, I turned and waved.

"You're welcome. Bye Cole."

At that moment, I realized I was not suffering, not inundated with my own pain. I was caring about somebody else's pain, and that momentarily erased all of my struggles.

☞

With one already down, I chugged another nauseating bottle of oral contrast. For those of you who are not familiar with this delightful substance, I shall describe it for you. It comes in a clear glass bottle, one that makes you believe that the milkman just pulled up in his horse and buggy, with fresh, ice-cold milk. It reads, "Barium Sulfate," aka, oral contrast. When you glance at the back, as if to read the "nutrition facts," you are informed that it can, interestingly, be taken orally, intravenously, or rectally. This made me appreciate the fact that I was *drinking* it. But—ahhh . . . the taste. At first whiff, it emits a vanilla scent, and you are momentarily tricked into thinking it is a sweet, smooth milkshake from your favorite fast food place. But as soon as the foul liquid slides to the back of your mouth, the chalky, bitter taste creeps up and hits you like Tax Day. Your mouth becomes pasty and dry, along with the glamorous bloating, stomach upset, nausea, dizziness, and loss of appetite. To add a cherry on top of the sundae from hell, you must fast before your scan. I pictured my belly, screaming for food, but only full of the sloshing, nightmare milkshake. So I had my moments of weakness and crabbiness, and I also directed several hateful comments toward the innocent glass bottle. But I eventually got it down, without any choking, gagging, etc.

My heart unexpectedly plunged down to my stomach and rebounded back up. I didn't imagine that the big sign that read "Cancer Center" would affect me in such a way. We were back in Santa Barbara after another long, tedious drive through the beautiful hills (just kidding). This time, we had Gramma Johnson along for support.

Entering the automatic sliding door into the cozy, inviting waiting room, Mom checked me in, and, just as I began to enjoy a magazine, they called me back. Mom and I were escorted down a long hallway, and I, although it sounds silly, was fascinated by the bright green carpet. We arrived at a small room that was composed of a counter, a stretcher-like bed, and a chair squeezed into the corner. A friendly man helped us get settled and turned to me with a grin.

"Can I get you a warm blanket?" he kindly offered.

Giggling with glee, I was unable to resist.

"That would be wonderful . . . thanks," I chimed.

Those warm blankets became my absolute favorite part of being in the hospital. Those toasty, comforting, heavenly blankets made me want to splurge and buy a warmer for myself. When he returned with not one, but two steaming blankets, I just about melted into my chair. I had died and was at the pearly gates for sure.

"Thanks warm blanket man," is how I remember thanking him.

And from then on, good old Luis from the Cancer Center was known as Warm Blanket Man.

They dug in my arm, like two gold miners, until finally they struck a vein . . . only it was a *blood* vein. The fluids began to drip, and I relaxed back into my chair.

"I'll bring you another blanket," Warm Blanket Man comforted.

Oh my gosh. He was my hero. Before long, another man, Ed, walked in and set a small, metal canister on the counter with a clunk. He explained to me that it was Fluorine (F-18,) a radioactive sugar compound which, after being injected into me, would create hot spots. It detected rapidly dividing cells and tissue by lighting them up on the scan. Allowed to hold the canister, I was astonished to feel how much it weighed. The heavy metal is used as a protective barrier between us and the radioactive solution. This radioactive solution had to circulate in my body for at least forty-five minutes, and I had to move as minimally as possible.

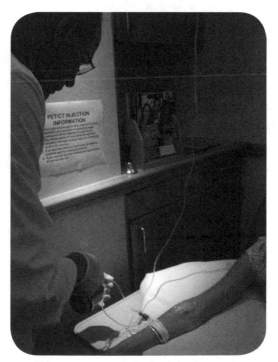

Ed corners my vein in the injection room.

So Mom and I sat there and talked for a little while. Then I stared at random objects. I specifically recall a certain square on the roof. It was different from all the rest. The vent on the ceiling was also a point of interest. Then, suddenly, something strange and unexplainable happened. This may offend some of you out there who are straightlaced, so my apologies to you. I became gassy. *Soooooooo* gassy. I swear on the Big Book of Farts that that was the gassiest I have ever been in my entire life. Within moments, Mom and I were in hysterics. Each fart brought on a whole new wave of belly laughter and silly jokes. It really wasn't *that* funny, but for some reason, our laughter was endless.

"What did they put in me?" I joked sarcastically, as we instantly collapsed into incessant giggles.

Both of us look back on this moment as a gift from God—the gift of laughter during that scary time. And yes, God's grace can even shine through farts.

The CT room was dark and somewhat damp, or maybe it was just my chills. I'm not sure. I was reacquainted with the giant doughnut I had met previously. And this one, just like the other, was disappointingly not the maple-glazed, rainbow-sprinkled delight I had hoped for. I changed, got on the table, and prepared for the journey through the doughnut hole. The extremely kind technician described all that was going to take place. After receiving an initial CT scan, I was to begin the process of the PET scan. The PET scan would take pictures of six different chunks of my body. Beginning at my toes, it would take nearly an hour for it to finally reach my head. We had to know how much things had spread, how serious things were, and the depth of the doo-doo I was in.

My entire body tingled with a warm sensation, and the room whirled around before my eyes. I felt like I was peeing in my pants, but all of these were common side effects of the dye that raced through my veins. With the CT out of the way, and the yucky effects subsiding, the machine was reset and the PET scan began. It was a long, tedious process, one that could bore anyone to death. Having so much time, lying there on that table, I began to get worried and anxious about what it might show. Bzzzzzz. The table moved a few inches, and the next phase began. What would they find?

Becoming overwhelmed, I tried to get the feeling back into my arms, hands, and fingers. I wiggled them frantically, even though I was instructed to keep perfectly still. My arms, which had been placed high over my head for nearly 40 minutes, were asleep so badly that they hurt. At one point, I could've sworn I was touching one hand with the other, but I couldn't feel a doggone thing. I was thoroughly convinced I would never be able to move my hands again, and the doctors would have to amputate. I tried to focus on something, anything else.

Bzzzzzz. Phase 3. This was exasperating. I counted the dots on the speaker that was mounted just above the opening of the tube. There were 123. Then, a song popped into my head. It is from *SpongeBob*, and it is titled "Best Day Ever." Closing my eyes, I began to sing silently, truly pretending it was "The Best Day Ever." And somehow, that silent song overpowered and drummed out the monotonous hum of the Monster Doughnut.

It seems silly now, but at the time, all I could think to do was repeat, "It's the best day ever, best day ever!"

The sun began to sink into the horizon as we left the Cancer Center. I had completely lost track of time, being in the windowless halls and dark, clock-less rooms. I felt like I had been at some sort of sick Disneyland, getting thrashed around in a futuristic world like Star Tours for five hours. Starving and exhausted, I dreamed of nestling beneath my soft, pink bedcovers.

THREE

THE FOLLOWING TUESDAY, we met with Dr. Tamir Keshen, a pediatric surgeon specializing in minimally invasive procedures. Within milliseconds of meeting him, his glowing warmth and toothy smile lifted my soul out of the depths to which it had sunk. We had opted to go forth with a biopsy, and this appointment was scheduled to discuss the matter. Dr. Keshen was fairly new to the hospital, but his intelligence and expertise were already highly respected by fellow staff members, as well as patients. I got the whole package, an excellent guy and a highly knowledgeable doctor. He resembled a bear to me, because of his tall, giant, yet gentle appearance. Behind his square glasses, his squinty eyes smiled with sweetness.

However, the twinkle extinguished as he brought on some unfortunate news. My soul began to settle back down as he gave us the clear facts. The mass sat on my airway, with the weight of it creating a large amount of pressure. Both Dr. Dan and Dr. Keshen were greatly concerned that, if put under general anaesthesia, my airway would entirely collapse. Just the thought of being completely unconscious, unable to breathe, ironically made it so that I couldn't breathe. I peeked over at my mom and dad. Mom looked pale. Dad looked frustrated. Dr. Keshen shrugged his shoulders and gave us a look of empathy.

"I don't feel good about doing it. I won't do anything I'm not comfortable with," he stated truthfully.

It was quiet for a long, awkward moment, and he then began to explain alternative choices. Innocently, I stared down at my pink Converse sneakers and wiggled them nervously. The only option was to put me under lighter sedation and to keep a very close eye on my vital signs. By the look on everyone's faces, I knew it was risky, but what else could we do? I, again, felt entirely helpless—a slave to my own body. We scheduled the biopsy for that Thursday, all too soon for me. But as I shook Dr. Keshen's hand and said good-bye, I put all my trust in him. God's light shone through him, telling me everything would be alright.

Wednesday was a day full of anxiety, and my mom and I strung up Christmas lights to distract our minds from all that burdened them.

I specifically remember thinking, "This might be the last fun thing I do for awhile."

My brain, a rotten grapevine, could not wrap around the stake of reality. I floated in between Earth and some horrible place. We finished stringing the lights and clicked them on. They looked beautiful, like a fire in life's cave . . . how symbolic.

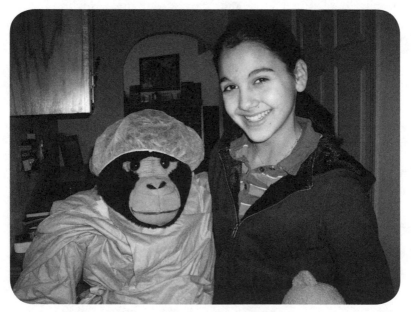

Antonio and I prepare for my first biopsy.

It was early, too early. I believe it's inhumane to get out of bed when it's so dark that you think you never went to bed. Not cool. But there I was, with my giant stuffed gorilla, Antonio, and bags under my eyes so big I could have packed for a weeklong cruise. Ding! The elevator made the butterflies in my stomach flutter as it jolted to a stop on the fifth floor. My mom, dad, and I waited, and before long, a nurse hit a large button on the wall, opening the huge doors into the world of pediatrics.

I kept my eyes fixed straight forward, avoiding looking into the rooms for fear of what I might see. I used to be scared of hospitals; I'm not exactly sure why. I guess I never had the inner strength to see someone in a rough state. That, as you can imagine, has changed dramatically. After checking in, we continued down the hall. It was lined with an underwater, dolphin wallpaper border that, if you stared at while walking, made them seem like they were swimming. As the nurse took a sharp right into my room, I couldn't help but wonder if I would have a roommate. I imagined the nightmare neighbor, moaning, screaming, puking.

My blood pressure returned to normal once we entered the empty, cozy, child-friendly room. A perfectly made hospital bed sat at the base of a large window that looked out on what seemed like all of Santa Barbara. A stuffed dog rested on it, waiting for me . . . I was touched. I sat on the very edge, thinking it was too creepy to lie in, or, in fact, get comfy on whatsoever. That would mean I was sick . . . *me*, sick in the hospital. I just couldn't bring myself to do it.

I was then asked a multitude of embarrassing and degrading questions.

"When was the last time you had a bowel movement?"

Yippee, my favorite. I chuckled. It wasn't exactly something I kept a chart on. Slipping into a gown, I wished I had about four more arms to help hold it up. Obviously, indecent exposure was not a serious crime here. Then, the waiting game started. I wasn't quite sure what I was waiting for, and, to be honest, I just wanted to get it over with. But the awesome view and the bright, sunny day that greeted me from the other side of the imprisoning glass made the time tick by. The clock's hour hand crept around, tickling its number face.

Also during this time, I was introduced to Jaynie, a beautiful lady who I now have the honor of knowing. She is the type of person who walks into a room, and everyone has absolutely no doubt that they are special and unique. Her illustration of selfless qualities makes her a prime example, and role model, for all human beings.

After Jaynie introduced herself, with the title Child Life-Specialist, I remember thinking, "Wow, this is actually your *job*—to make kids like me feel loved and cared for?"

I was fascinated with the fact that you could get paid for cheering people up and was convinced that it had to be one of the coolest jobs ever. My nerves began to settle as she gingerly consoled me and asked how I was feeling.

"Have you ever seen the OR before?" she inquired sweetly.

"No," I replied honestly, my foot shaking like it always does when I am uncertain about something.

"Would you like to see some pictures?" she offered.

Pausing for a moment, I softly answered, "Sure."

In a flash, she was out the door, and she reappeared a few seconds later with a large, white binder tucked beneath her arm. She enthusiastically plunked down right at my side and, like wings unfolding, the binder spread out across our laps.

"Now, when you go in, you'll see lots of things, and there will be three or four nurses in this area," she said, pointing to a specific spot in the picture.

"Your anesthesiologist will be standing here . . . he's the one who will be looking after you the whole time."

Smiling with appreciation, I was grateful for how much she cared about my comfort. We continued looking at the entire book, and as we sat together, my heart reserved a larger and wider spot for Jaynie, my new buddy.

The time had come. I heard the squeaky wheels even before I saw a man with a stretcher pull up to my door. I was relieved and ready, but jittery and procrastinating. I went to the bathroom one more time; funny how we overlook the simple things, like going to the restroom before surgery. Realizing how weird the patient ID tag around my wrist looked, I gave in and crawled under the starchy, white sheets on the stretcher. I had made a big step toward grasping the tough reality. Mom and Dad walked alongside as I was wheeled up, down, here, there, and everywhere by Joe, a great guy who became my personal driver, if you will. I cracked a smile . . . it was kind of fun. But my self-pity got in the way. I felt so screwed up.

Probably one of the weirdest things is having people stare at you as you roll by. They hesitantly peek, as though they're expecting a mangled, undistinguish-able thing to roll past. They sure did get a surprise when I went by, smiling and waving at them. Yeah, I milked that stretcher ride like Miss Pepperoni in the Parade of Pizza. We pulled up to a humongous door, it splitting as Joe pushed a Paul Bunyan–size button mounted on the nearby wall. Once again, a whole new world was revealed—the planet OR. It must have dropped about fifteen or twenty degrees when we entered the pre-op area, and I snuggled in deeper under my blankets, trying to shake off the uncomfortable chill. Lying down, I was unable to see the schedule board, but Mom told me later what it read. In big letters, my name was written on it like the Catch of the Day, battered, fried, with a side of slaw and unlimited soda refills . . . nah, just kidding.

It read, "Melinda Marchiano—Anterior Mediastinal Mass."

Mom confessed to me that when she saw that board, every ounce of warmth exited her body. It was chilling. Maybe having a visual idea of my situation in words, let alone scary, long, unpronounceable, medical terms, was just all too real.

A small, separate room branched off the hallway, and I distinctly remember Joe and me crashing into the wall as we jammed through the narrow doorway. Poor Joe took some major teasing for that one. As soon as we assessed the dam-age, and tucked into the closet-sized room, two nurses and an anesthesiologist walked in. The man was Dr. Willsey, a skilled sedation artist we requested for all my future procedures. We all knew how dangerous and daring it was to per-form the biopsy, but judging from Dr. Willsey's face, it was a cakewalk, a stroll in the park.

With calm, eloquent, and controlled words, he explained, "I'm going to keep you at a nice, happy place the whole time. I'm aware that there is an issue with the weight of the mass, so I'll just stay within the ideal range."

Great! I was convinced, never having been under anaesthesia before. He made it sound like a night's sleep in the Garden of Eden. Despite being hesitant and weary about my first experience with sedation, I couldn't help but feel some-what of a weight lifted off my chest . . . no pun intended. The wheels turning in my head burned with curiosity. I wondered, in that one moment as I drifted into unconscious darkness, if all the pain and the suffering would melt away. Would I finally get a moment—even a second—of peace and tranquility?

Looking innocently at Dr. Willsey, I thought, "Okay, you just do your thing, Dude."

The bright and colorful surgical cap that Dr. Keshen donned caught my atten-tion even before he did. It had SpongeBob and his pink, chubby friend, Patrick the Starfish, all over it. Between that and the huge smile that spread itself across his blushing face, almost all of my tension was shed, like a python revealing its new skin. He, again, sweetly and delicately described the procedure.

"We are going to make at least four passes," he said matter-of-factly.

He then went on to explain something about "firing the gun," which I tried to visualize as a pleasant experience, but I failed pretty miserably. Getting some-thing fired four times into my chest wasn't exactly on my Bucket List. Anyhow, when there was nothing else to be discussed, there was another very awkward, entirely silent, moment. I could sense Mom and Dad knew that it was time for me to go, but they wished it wasn't so. I understood . . . I felt the same way.

Mom gave me a kiss, and Dad gave me a pat, with a "Good luck."

I sure hoped that it didn't depend on luck.

An IV had been somewhat easily started, after the nurses finally cornered and stuck one of my unruly veins. The giant sloshy bag of pre-op fluids drained into me. Dr. Willsey approached, a syringe steadily gripped in his right hand.

"Okay, here's the happy juice," he assured quietly.

I felt utterly powerless as I watched him gradually push until not a drop remained. The stretcher creaked, and I was rolled toward the OR. Suddenly, the sedative hit me like a sixteen wheeler. Instantly, my vision blurred over into a blinding snowstorm, a winter not-so-wonderland. All of Jaynie's pictures came alive as I rode on my stretch limo into the actual operating room. The huge lights above me spun, three UFOs hovering in the dark sky. Someone placed an oxygen mask on me and all turned black as Dr. Keshen and Dr. Willsey worked diligently, collaborating and combining their brilliant minds. It was not until months afterward that I read my first biopsy report. Here's what it said:

> The findings are those of a dense fibrotic background with a poorly preserved infiltration of polymorphous lymphocytes including a background of prominent plasma cells and eosinophils. There is a large 12.5 x 7.5 cm mass that was surrounding the trachea and compressing against the carina as well as the mainstem bronchi.

The world was strange and distorted, almost alien, as my eyes—two tiny slits—were reintroduced to planet Earth. The faces of the nurses were fuzzy and warped, and I distinctly remember one of them jamming a straw into my mouth. Ugh. Thinking back to my iron supplement days, I cringed. I despised straws. Taking a tiny, pitiful sip, I felt the cool water slide down my throat and revive me to some extent. Dr. Keshen retrieved my parents from the waiting room, and they both stood close by as I awakened.

"You did great," Mom told me.

I smiled. I hadn't done anything, but I appreciated her kind words anyway. It was a long time before she told me what Dr. Keshen had shared with them.

"Usually, when I see kids like this, it's when they're in the ER, and they can't breathe."

To this day, I still take a long, deep, grateful breath . . . because I can. It is quite appalling that, as I slowly suffocated, my health insurance company insisted that "medical necessity was not established" for my care.

"America's health care system is neither healthy, caring, nor a system." —Walter Cronkite

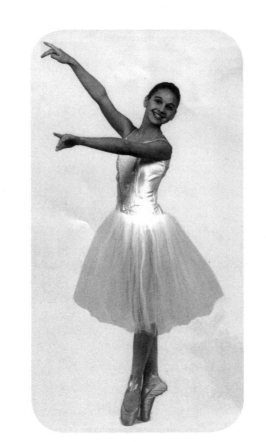

Nutcracker 2007.
Photo by Heidi Gruetzemacher, Photoworks Frame Gallery.

FOUR

THE BEAUTIFULLY HAUNTING "Waltz of the Snowflakes" music blared as I leaped onto the stage. I looked my part: ghostly, snowy white and becoming more so with each passing day. It was rehearsal week in the theater, and my chest ached, still sore from surgery. Plastering a *Nutcracker* smile across my face, I made it through yet another run-through. I always somewhat doubted whether or not I'd survive the marathon six-and-a-half-minute "Waltz of the Flowers," but I somehow found myself back in the dressing room, the potent smell of hair spray making it hard for me to catch my breath.

To be entirely honest, I'm not sure why I kept dancing during this time. Evoking memories of that stage during my eventual cancer downfall boggles my mind. But despite the fact that I struggled constantly, and it probably tore me up physically, I wouldn't have had it any other way. At moments, the frustration of trying so hard, but being so weak, got to me. I cried almost every night. My heart, an incessant waterfall, poured out deep feelings to my mom. She never failed to sit and listen, holding my hand so tightly that I knew she would never let it go. Thanks, Mom.

An uneasy feeling lingered within me the day we returned to the clinic for my biopsy results. Mom wore a strange face, one that looked different from any other I had ever seen. Breaking out in a cold sweat, I crammed my bottom next to Mom's in the big, square, pickle-colored chair. It seemed like we waited an eternity before Dr. Dan's familiar face popped in the door.

"Good morning, young lady," he recited eloquently.

"And how are you feeling?"

Firmly shaking my parents' hands, he pulled out a tiny toddler chair that stood at the nearby play table. As if he did it every day, he casually leaned back in the midget-size chair. Giggling, I watched as he tried to situate himself on the terribly uncomfortable seat. Dr. Dan has always been one to go to great lengths to make a child smile, even when that child is barely able to crack a pitiful grin. Like a bird on a telephone wire, he balanced there as he began to speak, or shall I say chirp. I cannot remember exactly what he told us, but I vividly recall my face getting hotter and hotter, until it felt like I was a lobster freshly plucked from a table-side aquarium and dunked in boiling, scalding water.

He informed us that the biopsy had been unsuccessful, and we then had two options. My mass was a rock, literally. It was an impenetrable blob of dense, fibrous tissue and who knows what else. We could either opt to just start treatment, or we could choose to have a second, CT-guided biopsy performed. Pointing out the pros and cons of each decision, Dr. Dan addressed the importance of finding a diagnosis.

I made up my mind quicker than Einstein doing an addition problem. I wanted to go for the second operation and, hopefully, finally, know what was making me feel so terrible . . . so . . . dead. It had become my enemy, and I had to find it and kill it, before it overtook and killed me. I wanted a name for it, one that doctors would recognize at first glance and, more importantly, know exactly how to treat. It is so strange to have an invisible monster, and enemy, tormenting your every moment. It ate me up physically and emotionally. The beast was within me . . . it *was* me. And whatever I had to endure, I was determined, with every fiber of my being, that I would conquer it. But the game of one on one was barely a minute old, and so far, I was losing.

The numbers and variables flew off the page at me as I completed my math lesson. Just then, Mom entered, the phone pressed against her ear.

"We're supposed to be there right now," she told me, her eyes wide.

She finished her conversation, and when she hung up, she replayed her talk with Nanci, the office manager at the clinic. There had been a slight communication mishap in all the chaos . . . they never called to tell us when my surgery would take place. While I peacefully slept, Dr. Willsey, and many others, waited for me to arrive nearly a hundred miles away.

Oops. A gut laugh broke out from both me and my mom. It was pretty funny. They called everyone but the patient. The biopsy express definitely couldn't pull out of the station without me. It was hysterical. But then, reality set back in, and Mom asked me what everyone else at Cottage Hospital wondered. Did I still want to come in? Mulling over the decision in my head, it rolled back and forth like an anatomical pinball machine. I slammed my math book shut . . . I was going in.

There I was, back on the stretcher, being rolled down the long, endless hallways. It was happening all over again. Staring at the little dots on the ceiling, my mind was a million miles away. Before long, I saw a familiar sight. The oxygen mask closed in on my face, slowly sucking me into an unnatural hibernation. With a CT scanner as my den, I slept, and silent prayers fluttered out of my heart and soared up to the heavens. Would we finally get a diagnosis . . . or would I be disappointed yet again?

☞

"I hope he took a nice big chunk out," I chuckled, observing the black-and-blue incision below the newly healed cut from my first biopsy.

It was the day after the procedure, and Dr. Dan informed my parents that he was almost certain that diagnosable tissue had been harvested. I was happy we had chosen to go for the second attempt, and besides the fact that I was in quite a bit of pain, I was in fairly good spirits. But I had to remain patient and go easy on myself—the two hardest things for me to do.

☞

I checked my incision. Okay . . . no blood, cool. My chest hurt pretty badly, like I split myself open where the doctors had. Picturing blood all over my pure white, sparkly *Snowflake* costume, I monitored my incision frequently. Although nothing was going to happen, I still peeked down the front of my long, elegant tutu often. Others probably thought I was a weirdo. With the famous *Nutcracker* music blasting, I made a grand, leaping entrance. Mom sat in the audience, holding her breath.

She later confessed to me she was scared out of her ever-loving mind, thinking, "I hope she makes it."

Her awe and disbelief that I was actually dancing only two days after my second surgery were equivalent to her worry and concern that I would pull through the show. Mustering up every microgram of energy I could, I channeled it all into my on-stage performance. Then, collapsing into a creaky dressing room chair, I sat and waited, hoping I could pull some energy out of somewhere . . . anywhere.

Throughout the entire *Nutcracker* process, I missed one, at most two, rehearsals. Replaying it all now, I'm not sure how, or even why, I pushed myself like that. It nourished my spirit to dance, yet it slowly destroyed me physically. But thinking it over, I know for a fact that I would not have changed a thing.

Like my mom and I always say, "Everything happens for a reason."

⌒

It was December 18, 2007. Strangely enough, I do not remember this day as well as I should. Only bits and pieces float in my mind, surfacing once in a great while before settling back down in the depths of my brain. I recall it as just another day in which I struggled with my health. But then . . . the phone rang. You have probably all heard the different ring your phone makes, the one where it screams to be answered. That's what it sounded like as Mom raced to pick it up.

"We have diagnosable tissue," Dr. Dan confirmed.

My invader was Hodgkin lymphoma, a blood cancer that attacks lymph nodes throughout the body. If left untreated for too long, it would spread to bones as well as vital organs. My family and I were all relieved to have a diagnosis, and I felt like I had already won one tough, long, excruciating battle. I had a sense of pride and control . . . almost power over it. But looking in our bathroom mirror, I thought I was looking at a different person. I knew, deep down, I would have to endure so much more in my lifetime.

⌒

Staring at my pale reflection, I thought to myself, "Wow, *I* have a disease. I have a *disease* . . . me . . . *Melinda*."

Everything felt so weird, so out of order. My life was a stack of blocks, all askew, off center, and bound to tumble to the floor. I pictured myself as what I was before I got sick, and an eerie silence came over me. The girl with innocent, brown eyes in my basketball picture on the fridge had no idea what was coming . . . the path she was on. That scared me. Every time I saw "me," it was a new "me," sick "me." Hodgkin lymphoma had invaded me and violated me.

⌒

It suddenly hit me, as I looked at the clinic walls, that the days had flown by, the wall decorations having faded from Halloween, to Thanksgiving, to Christmas. Mom and Dad both gave me that "reassurance smile" that I can read from a mile away. But I confess, I shot the same look back. As we herded into a room, I realized that even Dr. Dan looked different, serious, and I didn't like it. I could tell I was going to have to lighten things up.

We sat down in three, neatly lined up chairs, with me in the middle, resembling a nervous visit to the principal's office. But Dr. Dan was no hot-blooded, ear-burning administrator. His compassionate eyes met mine. He educated us, with the utmost tenderness, all about Hodgkin lymphoma and what treatment would entail. Listening as intently as I could, I tried hard to clear the fog from my head. At times, I only saw his lips move, but I caught enough to get the gist of things. I had "Nodular Sclerosing Hodgkin Lymphoma." My CT-guided second biopsy report explained the procedure:

> Using CT guidance, a 17-gauge cannula was advanced into a large anterior mediastinal mass and four large core biopsies were obtained with the Inrad automated needle. The gun was fired approximately eight times, but half of these attempts did not yield any tissue. The lesion felt "rock hard."

Thankfully, my PET scan showed us that the cancer had not spread into my other lymphatic organs. I was well aware that a total infestation would have brought on grim odds. My heart leaped to heaven and back when Dr. Dan shared that my survival chances were a gratitude-wrenching 96 percent. And even if possible relapse occurred, I still had a very high recovery rate. A million pounds of weight seemed to melt off my parents. I could only imagine how terrifying it must be to know your child has cancer and not know if he, or she, will survive. I love you, Mom and Dad; you are so brave and so very strong.

We continued to listen with curious minds, Mom vigorously jotting down notes on her pad of paper. I knew that immediately after we reached home, she would be on the Internet, educating herself on every scrupulous detail. Dr. Dan specifically told her to research *children's* Hodgkin lymphoma, because reading about the adult form would be "frightening." I appreciated the way Dr. Dan helped my mom prevent a possible heart attack . . . she had enough stress already.

In children under fifteen, Hodgkin lymphoma makes up 5 percent of the cancers diagnosed in the United States. It is more common in adolescents, and it accounts for 16 percent of cancers in teenagers. Although it is found more frequently in boys, girls are more likely to have it between the ages of fifteen and nineteen. A lot of times, the tumor itself cannot be removed by surgery, as was my case. Therefore, doctors must use radiation, chemotherapy, or a combination of the two. It is tricky business. They must determine the minimal amount of treatment possible, reducing dangerous side effects, while ensuring the complete cure of the disease.

This is what Dr. Dan spoke of. This is also the first time he used the word "chemotherapy," his New Jersey accent giving it a unique sound. My heart, a hair-raising roller coaster, plummeted down and did a double loop before finally ascending to the top again. Suddenly, that "medicine" that "melted the mass" revealed its true identity. I was totally and completely taken aback. Me. Chemo. It was unreal, like a fairy tale . . . actually a nightmare.

I looked to my dad, his eyes seemed watery. Instantly, I could see it hit way too close to home. His dad, my grandpa, had received chemotherapy for a very rare blood disorder, but sadly, he passed away that June after a long, grueling battle.

My dad's face read, "Oh no, not my daughter, not her too."

It was quiet . . . too quiet for my comfort, and way too long for my comfort.

Breaking the silence, I asked, "Will I lose my hair?"

"Yes," Dr. Dan confirmed.

Whoa. What a concept. I pictured myself resembling ET more than my own family. The positive, comedic side of me could not help but break through the layer of seriousness that coated me.

"Well," I chimed, "I won't have to put up my hair in a bun."

That brought a much-needed laugh to the dismal room, with Dr. Dan's deep chuckle making me laugh uncontrollably. Once our momentary silliness ceased, we got back down to business. I had one more inquiry that was haunting my mind.

"Will I still be able to dance?" I questioned, my eyes donning a soul-twisting, puppy dog look.

The answer somewhat surprised me.

"For the most part, yes," he replied. "We have a young man who played football through treatment."

That's all I wanted to know. I was set . . . content, a whole and complete person. Imagining myself bald as a newborn, dancing in class, I wondered how the other girls would react. I pictured shocked faces the first time I returned to dance, no one being able to concentrate with me in the room.

Then, Dr. Dan's next comment woke me from my ballerina daydream. He wanted to start treatment Thursday . . . two days after Christmas. We could all tell that he wanted to start that instant if he could, but there was some figuring involved, and he claimed he wanted me to "enjoy the holidays." I greatly appreciated this, but I was pretty sure it was going to be the most miserable, painful Christmas of my life.

⌒

I leaned against Poppy's van, trying to soak up even one degree of warmth to comfort me. My Gramma was lining up "the cousins" outside for the usual session of Christmas photos. As Gramma called me over, I dreaded leaving my toasty haven. Obeying, I forced a painful looking, droopy-eyed smile that still sends chills radiating across my body when I see the photo. It stares at me on our hall counter, my face not just a pearly white, but a sickly, disturbing, grayish blue. What truly takes my breath away is the look in my eyes. Many would only see a girl excited on Christmas, but I see the deeper, more intense feelings of pain, hopelessness, and trauma. I couldn't believe how incredibly sick I felt. In addition, I had woken up that morning with a terrible cold, and my head and throat screamed at me, begging for something cool and soothing to ease the pain.

Sitting around the Christmas tree, I struggled to remain upright on the big red couch as the presents were opened. I tried my very best to act like I was okay . . . I didn't want to ruin the day for everyone. I was in self-preservation mode, chuckling with cues from everyone, but never really knowing exactly what I was laughing at. Dinner came, but nothing tasted good, a major frustration when talking about my Gramma's delicious holiday feasts. Not long after we had all finished eating, I glanced at Mom. She instinctively knew it was time to go home.

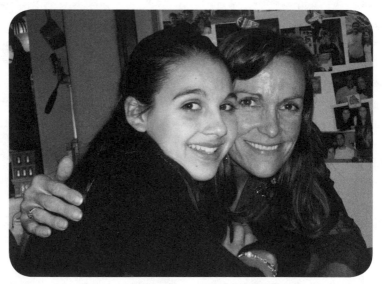

Christmas Day at Gramma and Poppy's house.

One of the most vivid, and well-remembered, events of my sickness is Christmas night. I sat in the bathtub slumped over, the hot water gushing out, making my head pound. The chills commanded my entire body, making me travel from

Antarctica to the Mojave Desert in a matter of seconds. My head hung so low, it nearly dragged in the water. And a weakness I had never experienced prevented even the slightest movement.

Closing my eyes, I could barely hear my shallow breathing over the roar of the water. Just then, I broke down, wondering why I had to suffer so much, why I was trapped inside this body that tormented me. Crying out desperate pleas to God, I asked for unrealistic things—total, instantaneous healing. That was the very first time that I questioned whether I would live or not. I truly, honestly, felt that it was the end. I imagined a giant headline on the front of our newspaper the next morning.

Nipomo Girl Found Dead in Bathtub on Christmas

I almost wished that God would just take me, free me and rid me of all the torture. Emotional breakdowns tear you apart—then somehow build you back up even stronger. I had no exceptions. Once my pity party had ended, I came to the conclusion that the only option I had was to fight and, in my mind, win.

☙

It's kind of odd that I don't remember the next two days. I was too sick, and too out of it, to function, let alone record the day for future book writing purposes. Mom called Dr. Dan to tell him that I was suffering from a bad cold which, according to him, would usually postpone the start of chemo—but not me. Dr. Dan wanted me in there . . . a discreet way of saying my situation was pretty urgent. A bone marrow aspiration and PICC line insertion were scheduled for Thursday morning, and that afternoon I would begin my first round of chemotherapy.

☙

The hospital had a different feel to me as I rolled swiftly into the PICU, or the Pediatric Intensive Care Unit. They had all the necessary equipment there to perform my procedures. The pungent smell of plastic tubing, alcohol pads, and non-latex gloves filled the air as we entered the cool, somewhat dim wing.

Focusing on staring straight ahead, I feared I would see some helpless child, who was barely hanging on, in one of the small inlets. I almost felt guilty being down there, like only if you were dying you had the right to be there, like I was rubbing it in their faces that I was healthier than them. I felt that I didn't really *need* to be there. My stretcher ground to a halt in one of the larger rooms, and I couldn't help but wonder if a child, or how many children, had passed away there. Studying the walls, I pondered how many kids the fish on the wallpaper had watched fight for their lives. I closed my eyes for a moment, saying the world's shortest, yet most meaningful, prayer for all who were there. I didn't know if it helped anyone, or anything, but it sure made me feel good.

Clenching my teeth, and nearly crushing my mom's hand, I grew tense from head to toe as the nurses attempted one of the worst IV starts of my life. But, with about two pokes in each arm, some major digging by multiple staff members, and sacrifices to the IV gods (just kidding), we somehow hit a nice, plump, juicy vein. Having gotten through what I thought would be the most difficult part of the surgery process, I relaxed a little bit.

Various nurses stuck heart monitor stickers on me. It tickled when they put them on; they were cool and gooey textured. With IV tubes and bags, as well as many heart monitor wires running here and there, I thought that, with any more equipment, I would be wrapped up like a mummy. So a note of surprise showed on my face as a blood pressure cuff and blood oxygen level reader were added to my collection of all things medical. A hospital sure does a great job of making you feel sick and messed up. Between the degrading gown and handles every two inches in the bathroom and the tangle of wires connected to annoying, beeping machines, you feel like a million bucks.

⁓

The man walking in nearly had to duck to clear the doorway. Dr. Pickert is his name, and he was the pediatric surgeon who would insert my PICC line. A PICC line is a long tube that is implanted into a vein, slowly fed up your arm, around the bend of your shoulder, and into a main artery near the heart. It would enable the chemo to circulate to all areas of my body in a very short amount of time.

I was now in the PICU, getting my PICC line put in by Dr. Pickert. I was "Picked" out. Also entering the room was Dr. Dan, who would be performing my bone marrow aspiration. They each explained, to my parents and me, the details of the procedure. Then Dr. Pickert confessed that, because of my unique case with the placement of my mass, he was having difficulty choosing between two types of anaesthesia.

One that he described, I have no recollection of, but the second option he told us about could cause "a little more dizziness" than the other. Nothing they discussed fazed me, and I trusted them completely and wholeheartedly. Anaesthesia was anaesthesia, right? Mom, Dad, and I left it in their hands and, once the more favorable had been selected, it was time to go. After getting a kiss from Mom and a hand squeeze from Dad, I watched them disappear around the corner.

Although alone in an unfamiliar place, with people I barely knew, I felt relatively at ease because of their kindness and reassurance. That long, fading feeling grasped my body, and the tiny pins and needles that prickled every inch of me carried me into a different land. I was asleep again . . . unchained and released from the confinement of my very own body.

⁓

"Are we done?" I mumbled indistinguishably.

I opened my eyes as much as I could, the towel over my head obstructing my view. I saw faint, blue blobs, nurses masked by an un-clearable blur. I tried to say a few other things to them, but my mouth was not capable of producing words. It was as if the cable connecting my brain and mouth had been severed, and it became frustrating. I then noticed the intense pain in my left arm, which radiated all the way up to my shoulder. I saw a strange contraption hooked on at the bend in my elbow and, when someone adjusted it, I grimaced in pain. I wondered where my parents were. We were done, right . . . right?

Suddenly, I heard Dr. Dan's voice as he reentered. Several nurses flipped me on my left side and began to scrub my lower back, practically my rear end. It hit me. It was not over. I had awakened right in the middle of it. Panicking, I shut my eyes, thinking I could make myself return to unconsciousness. But when I slammed my eyelids closed, I witnessed something just as scary. I was hallucinating. Just about every possible color flew around in a whirl, making me the dizziest I have ever been. It was dizziness that, if it was possible to die from dizziness, would have killed me. Also, for an instant, I saw the image of my mom, and I remember crying out to her in my head.

Thinking she was all too real, I screamed, "Mom! Mom! Come back! No, I need you!"

Her loving face was sucked into the spiral of flying colors, like a dust mite up into a vacuum. My heart couldn't take it. I opened my eyes once again, but terror gripped me. It was either the nightmare of all nightmares, or I was a spectator at my own surgery. I thought it was the end. I was almost positive that this was what it felt like to die. I was going insane, and nobody had a clue. Just when I thought I had nothing left, I remembered something. It was a Bible verse that my mom had taught me. She had said it to herself as she was in labor, giving birth to my brothers and me. Not knowing where else to turn, I turned to God.

"I can do all things through Christ who strengthens me. I can do all things through Christ who strengthens me," I repeated.
—World English Bible, Philippians 4:13

And that was it. I knew that no matter how painful or frightening it got, I could do it. I was in awe by how the verse spoke to me. I told myself that if we can do anything with the Lord's help, then we should not be afraid of anything. Pain is just pain, and God went through so much more of it for us than I can even imagine. God can do this, it is easy for Him, and He lives within me. Therefore, I can do this. No, I will do this. Just as the Spirit of the Lord empowered my soul, the big, long needle pierced my pelvis. The pain was so intense that I let out a bloody, yet silent, cry inside my head. It was like nothing I had ever experienced . . . or hope to experience again. And as Dr. Dan harvested my marrow, I talked to myself.

"The Lord is good. He is here with me," I remember saying.

I pictured Jesus, my Savior, taking all of the suffering from me, bearing it all himself. I knew that He would do this for me, and just the thought of it seemed to numb some of my discomfort. I am not sure if I finally returned to sleep or passed out from the pain, but after that, I have no recollection of anything. Maybe even the Lord, with his heavenly, pure anaesthesia, heard my prayers.

It was burning hot, and the room flew in all different directions as I awoke for the second time, this one thankfully *after* the procedure. The symptoms of a thousand cases of flu bore down on me with the weight of an earthmover brimming with a fresh, full load of dirt. With my fever skyrocketing, my body aching in every imaginable place, and my dizziness and nausea bordering on unmanageable, I thought back to Christmas night.

Only two days before, I had sat in the tub, helpless and weak. I had concluded that evening that it was the worst I had ever felt in my lifetime. Snapping back to my present state, I corrected myself. *This* was the absolute worst I had ever felt. I had one-upped myself, just not in the way one hopes to. I was monitored constantly and, being too ill and frail to open my eyes, heard and sensed the many nurses around me. I didn't like needing so many people to help me, but I was thankful they were there.

Just then, a sense and vibe in the room told me that someone I knew was there. I peeled up my eyelids, two five-hundred-pound garage doors that had to, unfortunately, be lifted manually. But when I got them opened, I was happy with what I saw. My brothers stood before me, little worried smiles plastered in their expressions.

"Love you, Quail," Nicholas said lovingly, using one of my many nicknames and terms of endearment.

He took my hand . . . it felt incredible. I knew that he would not let anything happen to me, and the comfort of his radiant, warm hand relaxed me. My eyes shut heavily. Remaining in that place for a short while, I focused on my breathing and grasping my brother's hand. I couldn't yet quite comprehend the events that had taken place during the procedures, but gradually, more and more memories that scarred me resurfaced.

Beginning to feel a tiny bit better, I gave glancing around another shot. I was pleasantly surprised to realize I was noticeably less dizzy, and relief permeated me as I gave my brothers a tiny grin. Suddenly, and without warning, I watched as Dean began to slide along the wall. He slowly slumped over the counter to his right before falling toward the floor. Nicholas and Dad lunged to catch him, and chaos broke out. Not able to see anything that was going on, I only sensed stress and urgency.

"Do we have an ice pack?" I heard a voice ask.

"Get some orange juice!" I recall another commanding.

All I could muster to ask was, "What's happening? Is Dean OK? Mom, is Dean alright?"

As I looked into her eyes, she gave me a fake smile, implying that he was fine. Somehow, I didn't quite believe her. What I heard scared me.

"Should we take him to the ER?" one nurse inquired.

Oh my gosh. What a disaster. My ears caught the sound of my dad, who directed a stern, serious tone toward Dean.

"Can you hear me? Dean, can you see me?"

Becoming a fraction more at ease, I heard Dean.

"Yeah, I can hear you."

"Can you see me?" Dad repeated.

"No, I can't see a *!%# thing."

Hey, watch it buddy. It doesn't matter if you're blind or not, this is a *pediatric* intensive care unit. Once ice was placed on the back of his head, Dean began to recuperate. Mom told me she knew he was entirely alright when he whipped out his cell phone to reply to a text. What did he type?

"I just woke up from passing out . . . what r u doing?"

"I'm not afraid of death, I just don't want to be there
when it happens." —Woody Allen

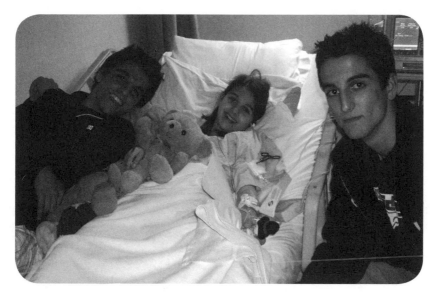

Dean and Nicholas offer bedside support.

FIVE

MR. FEVER PACKED his suitcase and went on a one-way trip to Iceland. Mr. Dizziness left the Merry-Go-Round Convention, and Mr. Nausea pulled into port, safe from the violent ocean storm. My vital signs were finally stable enough for me to return to my room. With a jolt, nurses unlocked the stretcher's brakes, and we started to roll. Everything may have been "stable," but I felt like I had been shot, punched, run over, and seared all at the same time . . . if that's even possible.

Wheeling back through the PICU, I felt more welcome there, more on the same level as those kids, but as I rolled out the giant door, guilt seized me once again. They couldn't leave. Heck, one un-plug and they would be lost forever. No matter how horrible I felt or how much pain I was in, I then always imagined someone worse off than me. It gave me a greatly needed dose of appreciation that I was going through a much-lesser evil.

As I mused over this, I again stared at the bland ceiling squares, like frosted-wheat cubes with cold milk and a big spoon. In my fascination with the cereal roof, I didn't see a wheelchair pull alongside my stretcher. It was Dean.

Cracking big smiles and shaking our heads, he asked, "How ya doin'?"

Pausing, I was in awe of our unique situation.

"I think the real concern here is you," I chuckled.

Ah . . . there's nothing like being concerned about another person to extract you from your own self-pity. We rode side by side in our sweet, new rides, occasionally giving each other a goofy, almost embarrassed smile. When we arrived back at Peds, we both parked, and Dean got teased mercilessly by Nicholas, Dad, and even the nurses. I giggled, my eyes barely open, like an alcoholic on free Bloody Mary night. Once I had exhausted every last drop of strength from my body, I fell asleep, the weakest I had ever felt physically and emotionally.

Pre-chemo fluids poured in, turning me into a peeing machine. My nurse, Cyndi, informed us that they must make absolutely sure that I was hydrated enough before beginning treatment. Frankly, if that was the case, I would have rather been dehydrated. Each time I shuffled into the bathroom there was a special "insert," I will call it, that had to be measured by Cyndi and tested for hydration upon my deposit. I appreciated the smiley face that was lovingly drawn on the bottom, but kind of felt bad for the guy. I thought that my end of the deal was pretty bad, but Cyndi's was pretty rotten too. However, she always wore a gleaming smile, her curly, reddish-brown hair making her all the more likable and adorable.

We were set to start chemo that afternoon, but with me still dehydrated and the chemo not even there yet, it became a matter of waiting it out. It had to have been a year since that morning. So much had happened, and I wanted to be done.

"Does this happen to other people?" I remember thinking.

For some reason, I thought that only I got tortured. The more I woke up from the anaesthesia, the more horrible I felt. Cyndi hit a large button on a remote.

"Bzzzzzz." The loud, industrial-sounding bed raised me into the air, like Frankenstein.

All we needed were lightning and some deranged person screaming, "She's alive! She's alive!"

Both Mom and Nurse Cyndi gave me goldfish and apple juice, but after I had consumed only three crackers and two sips of juice, I threw in the towel. To this day, I cannot even look at one of those orange fish with the cheesy smile or see a carton of apple juice without getting queasy. I have too many bad memories, all wrapped up in seemingly harmless, pint-sized packages.

⌐

At this time, I met my roommate, Alex. She was a sweet girl who, unfortunately, struggled with many health problems. Having been in the hospital for quite awhile, she shared her frustrations with being ill. I listened with a caring, compassionate heart, and then she asked about me and what I was there for. I explained that I had a huge mass, Hodgkin lymphoma, and I was getting chemotherapy to treat it.

Alex looked at me, her eyebrows raised as if to say, "Wow, I didn't realize how lucky I am."

I saw a sort of gratefulness, yet empathy, in her soft, twinkling pupils. Vanishing back to her side of the curtain, she reappeared just seconds later.

"Here," she said softly, handing me a tiny, smiling stuffed snowman.

Graciously accepting her gift, I thanked her. Then she got a piece of paper and started scribbling on it.

Giving it to my mom, she asked us, "Would you please give me a call, to let me know how you are doing?"

All of the air deflated out of my lungs, like a popped beach ball. Her kindness and care touched me. And besides giving her a teeny, pitiful smile and wave as she left the hospital the next day—that was the last time I saw Alex. Staring at that snowman, I gripped it tightly. Hours and hours passed into the night, and that snowman remained crushed in my left hand, my palm sweating profusely, but not letting go. If you happen to read this, Alex, I want you to know how much better you made that day for me, and that now, one year later, I am a cancer survivor. I pray you have won your own battles too.

꩜

It was pathetic . . . already wanting to be done so very badly, but I hadn't even gotten a drop of chemo. If it was possible to be at a negative step, I was there. With five kinds of chemotherapy, times four rounds, likely radiation, plus recovery . . . I was in for the long haul . . . the long, *long* haul. Just when I thought I couldn't wallow any deeper in my puddle of misery, Dr. Dan called a meeting in a small room across the hall from my little Chemo Hut.

I had to sit on the edge of the bed for awhile, summoning energy and strength to make it to a chair only ten feet away. I felt pitiful. When my rump touched down, like Neil Armstrong on the moon, I sighed—a long sigh of pride. But no matter how proud I was, that didn't mask the fact that I felt horrible, nor did it unhook me from the IV pole that slowly wheeled with me anywhere, and everywhere, I went. I can still hear the monotonous whooshing sound it made as I sat with my head propped on my hand.

My entire family was crunched into the small space, sitting on random chairs and stools. Dr. Dan pulled a rickety chair into the circle, his expression instantly setting a somewhat grim tone and feeling in the cramped room. He explained that it was The Chemo Talk, something all of "his kids" must hear. In other words, it was my right as a patient to know of all the possible side effects. With a heavy heart, and a soul of lead, I listened to him recite a long list of potential complications. They were as simple as a headache to as deadly as a heart attack. I was speechless.

Looking at my parents and brothers, their somber faces made an eerie sensation tickle my body. They had never looked so serious in all my life, and it was extremely frightening. I stared down at my PICC line. I wanted to go home. I didn't want to do this.

The chemotherapy, my lifesaver, was just as scary as my disease. I had a choice, but I didn't have a choice. I could either slowly suffocate to death or take on the possibly deadly effects of chemo and hopefully kill the Hodgkin lymphoma. I felt stuck, helpless, and hopeless. I thought that if the mass didn't kill me, then the chemo would. I was so confused, thinking I had to be the closest to death that I had ever come in order to be saved. It all didn't make sense to me. The feeling of uncertainty in the air was driving me nuts.

I couldn't help but think, "What am I getting myself into? Is this really necessary? Is this the only way?"

And even, "Would I really *die* if I didn't do chemo? Would it really kill me?"

The answer was, "Yes."

I finally realized, with my pee ready and my newly arrived chemo set, not to mention the 13 x 9 x 8 centimeter mass sitting in my chest, I had to do it. There was no turning back. Peering at Dr. Dan, my mom, and my dad, I felt a sort of thankful anger and frustration for them. They were saving me, but by torturing me and practically killing me. Uh, thanks?

At last, I made my way, slowly, back to my own room, struggling even more than before to put one foot in front of the other. I was so weakened and beat down emotionally from our conversation I broke down in Nurse Cyndi's arms. I didn't expect it, but I was just that scared.

Being so sick, crabby, and weak, I thought, "This is B.S.! I can't believe I just went and sat in there for them to basically tell me that I could just die from all this! Man, after fighting so hard!"

This buzzed around in my head like a swarm of angry bees. I continued to cry, and Nurse Cyndi comforted me.

"It's not as scary as it sounds," she consoled.

"People give chemo a bad rep . . . but it's really not too terrible."

She helped me back into bed as I wiped my tears away. I appreciated her kindness. She then disappeared, only to return minutes later, clad in a full, blue protective robe, goggles, and large rubber gloves. She held my bag of chemo, which illustrated a threatening hazard symbol on the side. All of the chemo nurses wear these alien looking clothes while administering chemotherapy to entirely protect them from it. I felt vulnerable, wearing nothing but a thin, ragged gown. Plus, that liquid she handled with so much caution, and avoided like the plague, was going to be put *into my body*.

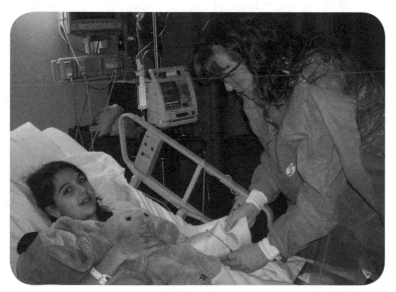

Here we go . . .

This was such an epic, major moment in my young life. As she attached and hung the bag on my pole, I knew I would have to fight, and I knew that the battle would be tough. The bag appeared to me as an army. I was afraid. It looked bigger and stronger than me. I think I was almost expecting a "one, two, three," but before I could sort out all of my feelings about the toxic liquid, I watched it drip into me. Holding my breath, a million feelings, emotions, and thoughts bubbled inside of me, like a pot boiling over.

My body is no longer pure; it will never, ever be the same.
My body couldn't make it on its own . . . couldn't survive.
I cheated . . . cheated on life.
I pray this works . . . that my suffering will be worth it.
I want to be normal.

"See," Nurse Cyndi told me. "It's not really that bad."

She removed her big blue gloves with a snap, and exited the room. I wanted to believe her . . . I really did.

I let my eyelids droop, as I began to feel the effects of the chemo. The poison didn't take long to penetrate my small body. This was the very first time I experienced how chemotherapy makes one feel, and I didn't care for it one bit. The nausea and dizziness exhaust you to the point where you can't even move a finger, and chemo delivers another unique feeling that is very hard to describe. It's a sort of "chemical feeling," like battery acid that races through your veins. I felt terrible, and as I write this now, recalling how sick I was, nausea and dizziness have returned to me. I only now noticed that, feeling so passionate about my writing, I am virtually reexperiencing it. Chemo may eventually leave your body, but it always stays with you.

The next time Nurse Cyndi returned, she held a small cup of pills. Oh, great. I became slightly nervous. I couldn't swallow pills. Having only taken liquid medicine for the duration of my childhood, I had never learned.

"Um, she can't swallow pills," Mom spoke for me.

"Oh, okay, I'll get some liquid," Nurse Cyndi replied, already halfway out the door.

Relief came over me like a tidal wave. Feeling the way I did, the last thing that I would want to do was sit up and get pills stuck in my throat, struggling to swallow them. So, I was very happy when I saw a little oral syringe appear on my table. Nurse Cyndi explained that it was my prednisone, and I would have to take 30 mg in the morning and 25 mg at night. Not knowing what I was doing, I opened my mouth cooperatively like a good little patient. Disgusting, acrid, vile, and nauseating do not even begin to describe liquid prednisone. I jammed fishy crackers and applesauce into my mouth, one more reason why those items have left my life menu. No person can truly grasp, or understand, just how putrid that medicine is unless they taste it. I'm making myself sick simply writing about it.

I knew then, I would be learning to swallow pills pretty darn fast. How I got it down, I'm not sure, but after I took it, my stomach felt like it had flipped belly up. It didn't help that my antinausea medication was not doing its job. Curled into a ball, I stared at the railing on my bed, and true misery began to set in. I shut my eyes, trying to let sleep take me away from my suffering. My IV pole, with its loud whooshing sounds, prevented me from resting. The noise—that began to drive me out of my mind—was a grim reminder of what I was doing. At last, a mess from the day, I fell asleep.

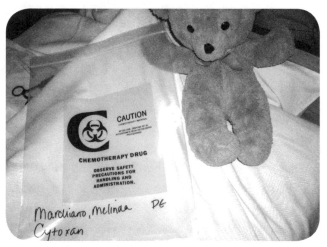

The visual definition of childhood cancer.

☞

I heard myself groan and pried my eyes open to look at the clock. Believing it was morning, I was shocked to see it was only midnight. Ugh. I tried to adjust myself to get more comfortable, but I found my weakness overbearing. I didn't want to move. Heck, I *couldn't* move. I let out another moan. My stomach hurt so badly. The pain was nearly unbearable, like barbwire was trying to be churned up and digested in my belly.

The cries and moans that escaped from my lips woke Mom, who slept on the fold-out bed nearby. As she turned to look at me, I blubbered and groaned in pain. I just couldn't help myself—that was one of the worst moments of my life. Mom reached for my small hand that hung, motionless, over the side of the bed. The tears flowing down my cheeks settled on my pillow, making it wet and soggy. I didn't believe where I was or how I felt. It was all too intense, too scary—too mind-blowing.

Lying there, I wondered if other people besides Nurse Cyndi and Mom knew of my suffering. While I sobbed, groaned, and experienced total and complete helplessness, people were sitting on their couches watching Jay Leno with a tub of Häagen-Dazs. My mind tried to grasp this concept, but it became too exhausted and failed. Words only from hell will begin to suffice in describing how I felt that night. The only thing that gave me hope was the warm, soft touch of Mom's hand.

I suddenly realized that I had to go to the bathroom very urgently. I told Mom, and she began to unplug and unhook everything that Nurse Cyndi had told us to unplug to go portable. As she ripped the blood pressure cuff off my arm, I tried to channel every last speck of my energy into sitting up. For a few minutes, I did the same as I sat with my feet dangling over the edge of the high bed, with my huge, no-slip socks barely scraping against the floor.

At last, I summoned everything I had and more, and we made it the twelve feet to the bathroom. When I returned, I was the most exhausted I had ever been. I "sprinted" for my bed, dreaming of falling asleep under the warm covers. I must have done way too much because, as I sat down, Nurse Cyndi grabbed my pink bucket, and I threw up violently. Darn. There goes my record. I hadn't thrown up for a few years. It was an *awesome* record, but one that was instantly flushed down the toilet when Mr. Chemo arrived.

Feeling slightly better, I settled back in and got reattached to all my equipment. Luckily, I had a new antinausea medicine, and it was beginning to make me nice and drowsy. Before I knew it, Mom was snuggled in my bed with me. She hugged me tightly and held my hand, the only gesture and symbol of hope and love in that dark, eerie room. We fell asleep in each other's arms, not having a clue what the future, or even the next moment, would bring, but not caring a bit at that time. And strangely enough, one of the worst experiences of my life held a special moment that I will cherish forever.

⌒

A giant, soft, smiling bear stared back at me as I awoke the next morning. It startled me somewhat, not having seen it before, nor expecting it to be there.

Feeling better, I was quite pleased when I had the strength to ask, "Mom, where did the bear come from?"

A smile erupted on her face, like Mt. Vesuvius, and she excitedly told me what had happened. While I was still in my own little dreamland, an elderly man with a giant sack had made his way into my room. He beamed at my mom with a grin that could only have come straight from God before displaying itself royally below his white mustache. The man volunteered for the Teddy Bear Cancer Foundation, a pediatric cancer foundation in Santa Barbara that we had yet to know of. Cheerfully, the man opened up his giant bag and extracted the biggest, most huggable bear. He looked from the chemo bag to me and watched it steadily drip into my frail, still body.

"I think you need this one," he whispered, as he placed the bear alongside me.

As Mom concluded the heartwarming story, I looked into the bear's eyes, and it looked back at me. I knew, then, that I was not alone and that so many people cared. That's it! Carrie. Carrie Bear. It was perfect.

⌒

The next few chemo-filled days, I managed the best I could. My nausea was finally controlled with just about every antinausea medication possible, and I even began to try to beat my previous no-throw up record. I received a total of five different types of chemotherapy on Thursday, three on Friday, and two on Saturday before I was discharged. Friday, I basically stared at my arm, watching it rise and sink on my stomach with my breathing. I tried to eat, but that whole department definitely wasn't happening.

However, one thing I did accomplish was to master swallowing pills. Well,

I shouldn't say "mastered," because several lodged in my little throat, making me choke. But sooner or later, with sheer determination, I forced them down. An extremely patient and kind nurse, Lisa, helped me in my pill swallowing endeavor. She taught me how to put the pill into my mouth on the back of my tongue, take a big gulp of water, tilt my head back, and slam it on down the hatch. I was very proud of my newly learned skill, and I think everyone else was proud of me too.

As I triumphed over the white capsules in my life, I was visited once again by my brothers and Dad. They had stayed overnight in a lovely, quaint hotel virtually across the street from the hospital. I soon learned that the Teddy Bear Cancer Foundation had provided their room, just one more act of generosity and compassion that made me love them all the more. Our family—helpless baby birds—had been taken under the wing of a loving, caring, and comforting mama bird. Lying in my creaky bed, I burst with gratitude . . . I felt so loved.

Nurses monitored my blood pressure very closely. This was because I was receiving my very last chemo in the hospital, Etoposide, which could cause my blood pressure to plummet unexpectedly. I rejoiced in the fact that I had almost made it through Round 1. But suddenly, I was faced with the fact that I still had to receive my final day of chemo at the clinic and repeat the process *four more times*. I had to survive a three-peat of stomach-ripping chemo, and to be honest, as I changed into my stinky clothes from the previous Thursday, I had many moments of doubt. It all seemed never-ending, like I was reaching for something that consistently moved away as I moved closer.

Trying to convince ourselves is a terrible thing, but that is what I had to do. Feeling half dead, I slumped into the waiting wheelchair and began to roll. Ugh. It was making me dizzy and nauseous, and I dreaded the hour-and-a-half trek home on the winding, scenic roads. I must have been a pretty bad distraction for other drivers . . . a pale, almost lifeless girl in the front seat of the silver Tundra.

I was rattled awake as we, at last, ascended our driveway. I was a wreck. Slinging my legs over to the side to get out, I nearly collapsed out of the car and fell into a heap on the pavement. But my dad was there, and grabbing my upper body and legs, he carried me into the house. I felt like I had left and gone to another world before suddenly and haphazardly being thrown back into mine. How I could leave our same house like I had, and come back the way I did, boggled my fragile mind.

Barely remaining erect, I studied my bright pink room, the multitude of stuffed animals eyeing me. I had just been lying in Cottage Hospital getting chemo pounded into me, and now, back in my own room, with my own bed, I felt out of place. Oddly, I had gotten used to that dark room, the invisible room-mate behind the drab curtain complaining day and night. I can still hear her screaming at her grandma, demanding Chex-Mix. Also, I had gotten used to the beeps, the grinding sound the bed made, and the loud buzz of my blood pressure cuff inflating at two in the morning.

My room was so quiet, and I closed my eyes for a moment, soaking up the silence like a sponge. Slouching over on my bed for quite some time, I peered around my room as if I had never seen it before. My body and mind were con-stantly taking in and processing new information, new environments, and it was extremely overwhelming. I was, officially, on maximum sensory overload.

Mom walked me to the bathroom. In three days, I hadn't bathed, brushed my teeth, or brushed my hair. I felt disgusting. As I sat on top of the toilet lid, Mom helped me peel the clothes off my back. When you're a thirteen-year-old girl, you don't necessarily want help getting undressed, but I just couldn't do it myself. I was naked, nauseous, and miserable.

I thought, "What if God takes me right now? Will I be naked in heaven? Wait! Let me put some clothes on!"

The instant my toe touched that warm, insanely body-melting, mind-numbing water, a tickle came over me. I immediately plunged into the tub, rejuvenated like I had never been before. It was a moment of my journey that I will always remember. Like a soldier injured in battle, I had returned home at last. As Mom washed me, I didn't even care that I was being bathed by my mom. I only rel-ished the amazing feeling of the warm water running down my back, alleviating all of my tensions. That night, I began to appreciate the smaller things, like a simple warm bath.

Being an active and outdoorsy person, I despised just *lying* there. Ugh. Frustration would escape, blowing steam out of the little outlets within me. I woke up in the morning to have breakfast, go to the bathroom, and pretty much fall back to sleep again. When I was more conscious, I flipped through the TV channels over and over, trying to find something even remotely decent. That was a battle in itself. During such awkward times in the day, nobody but little ol' me was watching TV. Sometimes I would turn it off and stare at things, letting my mind wander. Whenever I am in pain or discomfort, whether it be physical or emotional, that's what I do—stare. It helps me to focus, sort out thoughts, and push through whatever it is that I need to push through.

⌒

Pills defined my schedule, if you can call lying in bed twenty-four hours a day a "schedule." But seriously, we did have a Pill Calendar that Nurse Pam, from the clinic, had given us. And depressingly enough, this is how I recall my days:

Breakfast   **Snack**
3 Prednisone   1 Ativan
1 Ativan   1 Prevacid
1 Kytril

Lunch   **Dinner**
1 Emend   2 ½ Prednisone
1 Ativan   1 Kytril
                       1 Ativan

Having gone from absolutely zero medications to ingesting such a multitude, I was dazed, greatly overwhelmed, and kind of sick to my stomach.

It's terrible when you're just waiting for the day to be over, waiting for time to pass you by. Wishing I could push a giant Fast-Forward Button on the Remote Control of Life, I watched the clock's numbers slowly fade with the changing light of the day. Sometimes, waking up at seven, I was already anxiously awaiting bedtime.

My mom did everything for me: brought me my meals, bathed me, walked me to and from the bathroom, and just sat with me. Every so often, I would have to cry, and she was there within seconds to hold my hand. She would run her fingers through my hair, and I treasured that, not knowing when, or how soon, I would lose that too. I had my self-pity moments, but I soon realized they didn't do me any good and only wasted my energy. So many people loved and cared about me, and I knew they wouldn't let anything happen to me.

One of my problems was I was severely light-headed all of the time. My blood pressure was low, almost too low, because of a combination of chemo, medications, and my naturally slow, dancer heartbeat. When I sat up, my head would throb, and my vision would get fuzzy and dark. Almost every time I moved, my head would feel as if it was floating up to the heavens. I didn't like it. It scared me. But what could I do? I was in my body, and my body was devastatingly ill.

"I don't think of all the misery but of all the beauty that still remains." —Anne Frank

SIX

THE WORD HAD gotten out. Melinda has cancer. Like a wildfire, news of my illness spread like jelly on a crisp piece of toast. Cards began to pile up in the mailbox, surprising me every day. I would open them, and they would sing, "I Will Survive," or have a sweet, supportive message inside. Boxes would arrive at our doorstep, filled with PJs, blankets, stuffed animals, and fuzzy socks. Now I have a designated fuzzy sock drawer.

Another way for friends and family to check on how I was doing was through my CarePage. Robyn, the social worker at the clinic, told us of this online community.

My brother Dean referred to it as "MySpace for sick people."

Mom posted updates of how I was doing, and supporters left me caring messages. When I needed a little picking up, Mom would bring her laptop to me, and she would read me the loving posts from family and friends. It never failed to cheer me up and distract me from my pain.

Besides my pills, two other daily activities remain clear in my mind. One event was The Flushing of the PICC Line. As Mom sterilized the tip of my line with alcohol pads, I would bury my face in my pillow, fearing even a single whiff of the odor that I came to detest. After all of the air bubbles had been pushed from the small, plastic syringe of saline, it was securely screwed to the sterilized tip of my PICC line. The liquid raced through my line, preventing any buildup that could cause blockages. Next, another saline followed, and then came Heparin to finish the job.

Also keeping me busy, were the Neupogen shots that my dad gave me every morning. Just as I would down my last pill at breakfast, there Mom and Dad would come with my shot. At first, I dreaded that event of the morning, and I must admit that throughout treatment I didn't ever really get used to it. I recall the very first time I experienced that freakin' shot, an extremely painful occurrence I won't soon forget.

Amalia, my new home health care nurse, demonstrated for my mom how to administer it. She was a kind woman who would be cleaning my PICC line, drawing my blood, and giving me a checkup while I was out of the hospital. Studying the long needle, I knew I was in for some pain. However, I remained helpless, sprawled out on the bed we had made in the living room out of an old mattress and box spring. I was quiet, the way I always get preparing for any kind of discomfort. Listening to her instructions didn't help one bit.

"Turn it upside down and fill it up to this point here," she instructed Mom.

"Now you want to find a fatty part of the body. You can do it anywhere, but it hurts more if you do."

Oh great. She grabbed my thigh, pinching it into a tiny, pathetic fat roll. I wished I was fatter and wanted to tell her to wait, while I downed a few Big Macs. But before I could process my next thought, a shooting pain radiated in my leg, with my thigh as the epicenter. Then she started to push, and with each milliliter of that horrible stuff, it stung worse and worse. It was like a million bee stings, a belly flop from ten thousand feet, or forty-eight hours of tanning.

Saying my prayer, "*I can do all things through Christ who strengthens me*," I made it.

The long, drawn-out injection left me exhausted, sore, and already anticipating the next day's dose. But each morning, until my blood counts returned to normal, in came Mom and Dad with my shot.

It was strange having a nurse at home, and it made me feel like I was a thirteen-year-old girl in assisted living. Amalia would scrub my PICC line while I made faces to exhibit the pain I was in. Cleaning the hole in my arm with the tube coming out made me shiver and cringe. At first, I didn't enjoy having such a large medical "team," because it made me feel as if I needed a multitude of people to survive.

I very much desired to tell them, "I'm feeling a little better today. I don't need any of this."

But sadly for me, the numbers and test results showed them exactly how I was doing. My heart rate, blood pressure, temperature, you name it—they spoke for me.

One thing that surprised me, after returning home from the hospital, was how I felt about *not* being hooked up to nearly ten different machines. Initially, I was glad to be free, like a bird released from its imprisoning cage. But then, anxiety set in. I wondered if I *did* need to be hooked up to all those things, with cords and tubes at every angle. Whenever I had a wave of feeling horrible, I wondered what it was that was causing it.

Convinced that I should be displaying my vital signs at all times, I guess everyone else knew of my stability, but I did not. I only knew how I felt . . . insanely terrible. Lying in bed, nausea, shortness of breath, and unbelievable weakness tortured my body and clouded my mind every moment of every single day. Also, my body was penetrated by deep, deep pain from the Neupogen shots. My legs, arms, back, and neck all ached intensely. It was like someone had ripped the bones out of me, banged them around, and returned them to their proper places. It was a haunting pain that Tylenol could barely numb.

So all I could do was stay there motionless and trust: trust that the pain would go away, that everyone helping me knew what they were doing, and that I would eventually be the smiling, healthy girl on the fridge again. I began to sleep in my mom's bed with her while my dad bunked out on my temporary bed in the living room. We all agreed that it made us feel less uneasy. I was closer to her, and she was closer to me, just in case I needed something.

One night, I awoke to discover that I had to go to the bathroom, *really* badly. However, feeling so horrible and weak, I spent quite awhile figuring out just how urgently I needed to go. Walking to the bathroom seemed like attempting to summit Everest right then. So I just waited, awake, gazing up at the high ceiling. A short time passed, and I was *dying*. So, I finally accepted that I had to yank myself out from my mom's toasty covers and make the fifteen-foot trek to the bathroom. I flipped over, like a seal sunning itself on a warm day.

Gently tapping my mom, I whispered, "Mom, I have to go to the bathroom *really badly.*"

She must have leaped out of bed before she even opened her eyes, because she was around the other side of the bed and helping me up before I knew it. But unfortunately, being as sick as I was, I could not hold out till the bathroom. I will not go into detail, but long story short, sadly, we only made it as far as the shower, the peeling caulking vivid in my memory. I started to cry as Mom cleaned up; I felt terrible for her. Between my pain for her and my own pain, I could barely stand it.

"What's next, a diaper?" I thought.

Still sobbing, I must have told Mom a billion times how sorry I was. This was always her response.

"I love you. It's not your fault."

I have forever been one who is slightly—okay, really—hard on me, and I don't like to have to have my needs met by other people. But suddenly, I couldn't help being needy or dependent, yet I still fought it. Recovering somewhat from the ordeal, I noticed just how exhausted and fragile I felt. I softly shut my eyes, still crying a bucket of tears. I will never forget what Mom told me.

"I know it's hard right now, but guess what? At thirteen years old, you are going to be a cancer survivor."

Wow. It dawned on me. I had *cancer*. That was the first time that anyone, Dr. Dan, nurses, friends, or family, had ever used that word to refer to my illness. I think that it was probably avoided and aimed more toward Hodgkin. Hmm, that sounds like a cute little puppy with floppy ears, compared to "cancer." They probably didn't want to scare me, and I thank them for that. I knew I had cancer. I was getting chemo for goodness' sake, but never before had that word been directed toward *me*, describing *me*. And, from that point on, a little tape played in my head—periodically rewinding itself before repeating again:

"I have cancer. *I* have cancer. *I* have *cancer*."

Still, after all that, my very next thought was, "Are you sure? *Cancer*?!"

❧

Trying to fall asleep one night, I began to focus on my breathing. I tried to take a deeper breath, and it worked. And then I took a slightly deeper breath. That worked too. The tiniest tickle was felt deep down my runway, oh, I mean airway. When I took a breath, it seemed almost as if a portion of my trachea had never felt the cool air rush past it. Was it really happening? Was my airway opening up? Excitedly, I continued to play with my breathing, filling my lungs to the brim before gently blowing out. The tickle remained, and I described it to my mom.

"I have a whole new airway being born."

The strange sensation, deep within my chest, remained, and I didn't mind it one bit.

My appetite was, fortunately, increasing, most likely a result of my steroid medication, prednisone. Dr. Dan informed me that I would be hungry frequently, be moody, and that my body would puff up slightly. But still, even with his warning, starving, crabby, and looking like the Michelin Man wasn't exactly what I expected. I would get intense cravings, extreme desires for ice cream and cheese omelettes, among other things.

The morning after returning home from the hospital, the absolute single thing I felt like eating was waffles. Mom had a waffle iron out in two seconds, and she had never been happier to cook up a hot, steaming batch for me. I downed three waffles, an amazing feat for my chemo-scarred belly that had been nearly empty for three days. I continued to eat pretty well, thanks to my bitter, acrid appetite stimulant. Without my prednisone, I probably would have wasted away to nothing. Although food didn't smell the same, or taste the same, I especially enjoyed it when friends or family would show up at our front door with dinner. A surprise would be tightly wrapped under foil, still warm and fresh from the oven. Lasagna, casseroles, you name it—they arrived on our doorstep via loving arms.

Shortly after I arrived home, I received a visit from my Gramma, Poppy, Great-Aunt Ruth, and Great-Uncle Wen. I could see a strange look on their faces, as they rounded the sharp corner into the room. I almost felt embarrassed for being in the state that I was and thought that a "You Get What You See" sign would be appropriate. Watching them come closer, I pictured one of those cheesy soap operas. You know, one where the sick person lies in the bed, practically dead, while people come to see them one last time. It all seemed like a soap opera, depressing, and *way* too dramatic for my comedic flair. I was afraid I would not be treated like "Melinda" anymore, that things would be different between me and those who I knew. But I realized, quickly, that it was the same people I love dearly, and that they had come to share their love with me.

My Great-Uncle Wen and I have an ongoing joke, where I tell him, "I like your hair!"

I gently pat him on the head, while a deep, low chuckle emerges from his smiling lips.

He then turns to me, repeats the same hair-frizzing motion, and says, "I like your hair!"

We end up laughing together, each rubbing the other's head.

So this time, when he announced the famous line, I joked, "Enjoy it while you can!"

Laughs erupted from everyone in the room. It made me happy.

Hearing them try to catch their breath and contain their giggles gave me a feeling of purpose. I then began to realize that giving is a source of healing, treatment, if you will. I discovered that although I could get my health stripped away from me, nothing could take away the love I have inside my heart. Staring at their beaming faces, I saw something deeper. It was a cycle. They gave to me, and I gave to them. Our love circulated, like a never-ending pump, with more and more tender affection pouring in each moment.

Also, I began to realize that my situation created an opportunity for people to give. At first, I felt bad, and a little awkward, with so many people sending me gifts, making dinner, etc., but it suddenly occurred to me that they *wanted* to give, and *wanted* to help. It made others feel wonderful to do something for me and my family. And so, I began graciously accepting all of the love and assistance that flew my way, giving back to them the love in my heart they had planted there in the first place.

☙

On January third, I headed back to the clinic for my last punch of chemo for Round 1. Beginning to feel a tiny bit better, I thought of what a terrible, depressing thing that chemotherapy is. It shocked my body with a sudden surge, dragging me down to near death. And then, just as my body began to recover, it was a signal to slam me with even more chemo. Basically, they kept me consistently dying. As Mom, Dad, Dean, and I ground to a halt at the main entrance to Cottage Hospital, I honestly didn't think I could take anymore.

Shutting off the car, Mom gave me a look, as if to say, "Can you walk?"

I hung my head, sadly shaking it. I wanted to be able to walk so badly, but I knew that I simply could not. Dad hopped out of the car and came into view moments later with a wheelchair. Sadness overcame me . . . I could not even stand on my own two feet. When you're a teenager, at the prime of your youth, you should be able to run, jump, climb—whatever. But there I was . . . my legs two slices of Jell-O, not even able to hold up the scrawny, little weight of my own bony body. This only happened to old people, right? Yet, there I sat, living proof—thankfully—that anything can go wrong at any given moment. When I wasn't lying, I was sitting. When my bottom fell asleep, I returned to my semi-horizontal position. It became demoralizing.

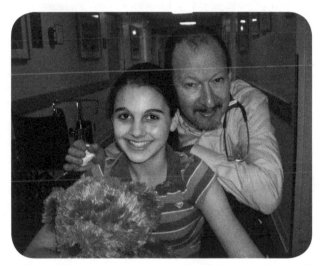

Dr. Dan and I stop for a picture as we roll down the clinic hall.

We wheeled into the clinic, and the smiling faces of Nurse Pam, Nanci, Robyn, and Dr. Dan filled my soul with a light, a ray of sunshine and hope. Even the clinic's other Nancy, who everyone calls Zippy, was there to greet us with her warm grin. As they saw my wheelchair, I instantly witnessed their expressions of sympathy. I have always pushed myself to do, and achieve, whatever it is I wish to do, so accepting the fact that I physically couldn't walk and had to throw in the towel was extremely hard for me. Borderline ashamed as I rolled into the treatment room, I took a single step up onto the long, hard table. Frustration clogged my mind. Why couldn't I *do* anything?!

"Walk! Walk, gosh darn it!"

But my anger turned to gratefulness as Dr. Dan reported to us that my bone marrow aspiration showed no signs of cancer. I then became ashamed of my anger. I had a lot to be thankful for, and I needed to acknowledge that. Although I was trying to maintain my positive outlook, it was quite difficult to think about the bright side as a small syringe pump began to reacquaint me with the delights of chemotherapy. I was getting more; I couldn't believe it.

With self-pity once again sneaking in the back door, I became suddenly distracted by a girl, slightly older than me, walking into the room. She filled the room with her shining smile and warm, radiant glow. Nurse Pam introduced her as Rachel, one of their patients who had beaten Hodgkin lymphoma about a year before. We shook hands, and I noticed her short, wavy hair. It looked cute. As I continued to receive chemo, she approached me, and we began to talk. She told a little about herself, and then we started in on a discussion of treatment and recovery.

"Poor Melinda here has had a tough first round," Nurse Pam empathized, flushing my PICC line with saline.

Rachel gave me a compassionate look. She had once been there. I could read it in her soft, brown eyes.

She looked straight at me and said reassuringly, "Don't worry."

Her calm, gentle voice was soothing.

"The first time is the hardest, and then it gets easier and easier with each round."

I believed her. She had been in my spot a year ago, and I trusted her completely. It is amazing how two strangers, people who have never met, can be instantly bonded by something in the world. Our lives are an intricate web of roads, each an option to go down. Yet, it seems to me that every single person we come into contact with is meant to be. Rachel and I are two humans, plopped down here on Earth, bonded by an unforeseen medical nightmare.

As she waved good-bye, I waved back, feeling like I had known her my entire life. I believe God placed her there that day to give me hope, determination, and courage. Looking to Mom, who sat in a little blue chair, I saw she had tears in her eyes, and that's when I realized that, I too, had eyeballs brimming with tears. I wasn't even exactly sure why I was crying. Rachel had inspired me, and her simply standing there, a happy and healthy girl, gave me a picture of my future. It gave me a goal. I was in awe of the way that God created a bridge for us and used one life to touch another.

Just as I was beginning to sense the "chemo" feeling once again, luckily, I had another distraction. Robyn entered with a large plastic box and a paper cup. I was curious, and intrigued, as she plunked down, table side, right next to me.

Printed on the box in huge, colorful letters were the words *Beads of Courage*. Her short hair bobbed up and down excitedly as she told me all about it. Cancer kids create a necklace by stringing together different colored beads that represent pokes, operations, ER trips, etc. She placed a long string in the paper cup, and then I began to make my selections.

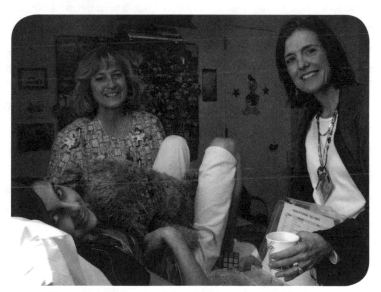

Nurse Pam, Robyn, and I pick out my Beads of Courage.

Slowly reaching for the bright green beads, I dropped them, one by one, into my cup—they were for tests. Next, I received white beads for days of chemo and yellow ones for days in the hospital. I added the pretty, dark blue beads, as they too joined the others. They were for clinic visits. Lastly, I acquired an orange bead for my PICC line, four tan ones for my biopsies and bone marrow aspiration, and black beads for pokes. As black began to drown out the other colors in the pile, I realized just how much of a pin cushion I had become. I already had quite a collection and began carefully threading them onto my big, long string.

Reaching for the letter beads, I spelled out my name before looping and adding the rest. Wow. It was already nearly half full, and I then knew why Robyn had given me such a long string.

My necklace is a symbol of what I had done and what I would do. I felt proud as it rested around my neck, each one of those beads telling a different story, a separate struggle, and an eventual triumph. It might be just a little necklace, but it means something so much deeper to me.

Nurse Pam appeared frustrated as she watched my blood drip, slowly, into the purple-capped vial. It was exasperating, lying there watching each tiny drop of blood create a teeny puddle in the bottom of the tube. For some reason, she couldn't draw labs from my stingy veins, and she had to resort to injecting me with a blood thinner. I had to let the thinner circulate in my body for a reasonable amount of time, so I mounted my wheelchair and sped down to the cafeteria to kill some time. Rolling up to the high counter, I pointed to an elaborate chef salad in a little plastic box. Lifting the glass door, Mom extracted it from the case, and we flowed into the checkout line, amid the sea of blue scrubs.

I crunched my lettuce, trying to taste something, anything. It was no use. The chemo was starting to overtake my body once again, and all senses became annoying, nauseating, and completely unappealing. But, like a robot, I repeatedly lifted the fork to my mouth, accepting the fact that I could not thoroughly enjoy it. My wheelchair sat in place of one of the table's chairs, and I examined the mass of doctors and nurses. Pagers were clipped on their hips, stethoscopes were wrapped around their necks, and the shuffling sound of those silly blue booties filled the room.

Suddenly, I caught sight of a familiar face. It was none other than Dr. Pickert, the doctor who had inserted my PICC line. He, unfortunately, opted to use Ketamine during my procedure, the sedation that I had reacted so violently to. By this time, I was punchy from the exhausting day, the chemo and meds making me drowsy and unpredictable. He was not within earshot, so I found words flying out of my mouth.

"Hey . . . Dr. Pickert! Nice call on the anaesthesia!" I asserted in a chemically induced stupor.

My family busted up while I, sarcastically, acted like I was going to read him out. When I couldn't keep a serious face any longer, I too broke into a drunk-sounding chuckle. Peering across the cafeteria, I munched my salad vigorously.

I had no bad feelings whatsoever for Dr. Pickert, and I never will, but it was just my nature to turn any situation into a laughing matter. I was drowning myself, and everyone else, in a pool of sarcasm.

I sighed in relief, as did Nurse Pam, when my deep red blood began to flow back at the clinic. However, I couldn't look at it for too long or I would risk getting woozy, with the possible consequence of losing consciousness.

It felt like heaven when I finally returned to the warmth and familiarity of our car. I was embraced by the giant, soft, fuzzy pillow that had waited patiently for me while I was inside Cottage Hospital. Feeling insanely queasy, I mashed my face deep within my pillow—it helped. Nearly in another pillow world, I thought about the road to come. Four rounds . . . *four* rounds of this. It felt like it would never be over, like I would spend my entire life struggling, fighting.

"One down, one down," I told myself.

Closing my eyes, I squeezed them shut as tightly as I possibly could. Somehow, it numbed the pain a little.

"Laughter rises out of tragedy, when you need it most, and rewards you for your courage." —Erma Bombeck

SEVEN

ONCE AGAIN STARING UP at our bland, white ceiling, I anxiously awaited the next checkpoint in the day. These "checkpoints" were anything that got me remotely excited, made me feel good inside, or at least distracted me from how I was feeling. The morning crossword puzzle, the mail coming, and when *Sponge-Bob* came on were all times that I looked forward to. But as soon as the puzzle was done, the mail was opened, and the *SpongeBob* credits rolled past on the TV screen, there I was again, lost and indecisive.

One particularly difficult day, shortly after my clinic chemo, found me scratching and scribbling at the crossword puzzle, nothing making sense. I gave up—my emotions a brittle twig about to snap. After my morning pills and shot, I snuggled deep under the warm covers, my mind wandering back and forth between the pain in my arm and the bitter taste of prednisone that still lingered in my mouth. Gasping for breath, choking on my own self-pity, I melted down like the polar ice caps. It wasn't fair. It all wasn't fair.

I gazed out our front window, my eyes capturing the bright, gorgeous day. Imagining myself sitting in the cool shade of the Sequoia tree after a long walk, I practically heard the birds chirping, the temperate breeze gracefully sliding past my face. The greater and clearer the vision became, the faster the tears erupted from my eyeballs. I struggled to evoke my "childhood" feelings—the innocent times that made me feel so alive, so in the moment. I remembered the sensation I used to get in the summertime, and I yearned to smell the sweet mixture of fresh-cut grass, along with chicken and garden vegetables sizzling away on our grill. I longed for energy and recalled when I would spend entire days playing outside.

☞

Dean and I, especially, would play silly games for hours and hours on end, exploring our acre lot each time with excitement, as though we had never seen it before. Cardboard boxes would transform into duct-tape-covered cars, tanks, and houses. Stuffed animals would go on daily adventures . . . each one whatever story our brilliant, young minds conjured up. Little Bear got lost in our "rain forest" bushes, or Teddy scaled the backyard wall like a rock climber. As far as we were concerned, fun was a renewable resource. Time flew by so fast and was filled with nothing but excitement.

We made a baseball diamond, precisely mowed on our lawn, where my brothers and I would spend the duration of many days, with teams of stuffed animals, all carefully set in their positions on the field. Grand slams, stolen bases, and the occasional brawl resulting from a bad call all composed our creative "script." The only thing that stopped us was when Mom would appear at the screen door with grilled cheese and a big, cold glass of milk. Worry didn't exist, nor did responsibility. Each day was a whole new bundle of fun, just waiting to be opened.

☞

Sadly, I failed in my attempts to bring back those incredible feelings—to experience them once again. It then occurred to me: I did not remember when I last felt normal, healthy . . . human. Father Time had fooled me and had pulled the rug of progression out from under me as I stood on wobbly legs. My face became red and hot, my tears feeling cool against my cheeks.

"If only for a second, *one* second," I thought. "I can relive before. If only I can be reminded of what it feels like to be well."

Mom rubbed my back. I had not seen her come in.

Through my desperate sobs, I spoke softly, "I didn't sign up for this."

I wondered, then, if I would ever experience pure joy and happiness ever again.

☞

January sixth was a small, itsy-bitsy victory for me. It was the very first night since December 26, 2007, that my head hit the pillow and did not stir until the morning sun kissed my face. Awakening more fresh and rejuvenated than I had in quite some time, I did a bed hop from my mom's to my dad's and got settled in for the day. I rarely shut my eyes, let alone went to sleep, during the day and therefore busied myself with various games and activities.

Nicholas plunked down on the bed, making me bounce, and asked, "Hey Mushy, you want to learn how to do the Rubik's Cube?"

I smiled. "Sure!" I replied. "What the heck," I thought.

My schedule was clear.

Studying the way my brother whipped it around in his hands, turning and twisting the bright colors, became somewhat disorienting. Within minutes, it was perfectly arranged, each color occupying its own side. Intrigued, I wanted to learn. Nicholas handed it over to me, and I aimlessly spun the cubes every way but the right way. But slowly, I began to complete more and more of it, as Nicholas taught me the vast array of moves and techniques. I was touched that he wanted to spend time with me, and I don't believe he knew what a bright spot in my day that he had made.

He helped me, quite a bit, to solve it the first time, but before long, I was a Rubik's master. Okay, maybe not a *master*, but to me, time didn't matter. When he left me with that little, simple cube, I solved it over and over and over again. The combination of accomplishment and distraction was perfect for me. Finally, my forearms and wrists burning, I settled down, still gripping the perfectly solved cube.

A couple of days later, I began to be relieved of the major weakness and nausea the chemo had dumped upon me. Although it was only to a certain, somewhat pitiful, degree, it was still a step toward improvement. I was more mobile. It was easier to walk to the bathroom and back. It's amazing that, at that time, I considered an ounce of strength "strong." Even though my "strong" was weak beyond belief for others, it was the power of an ox for me.

It truly goes to show that people's perceptions vary greatly in this world. We all think that there is a general and normal meaning for everything, but our views are so very, very different. One's "sick" might be another's "well"; one's "hate" might be another's "love"; and one's "poor" might be another's "rich." Likewise, one's simple task might be another's victory, like later on that same day.

The distinct hum of the mail truck grew louder, until I heard the brakes screech to a stop in front of our house.

"I want to get the mail today!" I said excitedly.

Eyeing Mom, I observed her expression. I detected a note of her feeling it was too ambitious.

But then I heard, "Alright, but somebody needs to walk with you."

Elated, my heart soared. I would get to go outside for the first time in a long, long time. Anticipating the incredible comfort and warmth of the sun on my face, I slowly made my way to the front door, careful to plant each step firmly. Dean walked beside me, holding my arm as if he were leading the blind. The unique sound of our door opening filled my ears, and I gingerly stepped outside, careful not to trip. Being erect, I was woozy and light-headed, but the smile that shone on my face did not reveal the slightest clue.

As we came out from under the eaves of our house, the world seemed to open up. I was doing it. I was walking. Dean kept a firm grip on my right arm, a symbolic bond between brother and sister. We traveled at a ridiculous pace, but neither of us cared. We almost seemed to glide along. The air smelled fresh, like barren winter blossoming into newly born spring. I heard nothing, for I was in awe of God's beautiful day and so focused on putting one foot in front of the other. I relished every blade of grass, each leaf that crunched beneath my pink fuzzy slippers.

After retrieving the mail, Dean and I started up the driveway. I felt extremely tired and knew that payback would be the rest of the day, and probably the next day too. But that was the last thing on my mind as I retraced my steps back to the house.

Suddenly, I had an idea. Breaking free from Dean's grasp, I turned on the turbo-boost. It was still painfully slow, but just enough to make my brother laugh in surprise. That tiny, three-second acceleration told him I was going to be okay, maybe not anytime soon, but eventually. It told him that, even though cancer had invaded his sister's body, it hadn't invaded *her*. My hand loosely gripped the door handle . . . a gratefulness and pride bursting within my feeble body, yet iron soul.

I must have been empowered by my daring feat that afternoon, because the following day, I tore off my pajamas and donned a T-shirt and sweats. It was practically PJ's, but just getting changed into something different in the morning made me feel less sick—not physically, but psychologically. The sensation of rotting away in the same pajamas for twenty-four hours made me cringe.

I was becoming an antsy little patient, a cheetah locked in a three-foot-by-three-foot cage. I was the cheetah, wanting to run as fast as I could, but restrained by an inhumane cage . . . my body. I had to do something, anything but lying there *all day long*. Opening and closing the chest of drawers in our hall closet, I ran across an activity book.

"Build Your Own Western Town," it read.

Hey, what the heck. With tape, scissors, and paper clippings, I sat in bed for hours, my bottom falling asleep until I could no longer feel it. Diligently, I assembled the buildings, carefully examining each adjustment I made. Something was so simple about sitting there, focusing on the little windows and swinging saloon doors. It didn't matter how long I took, I could re-tape the chimney forty times if I wanted to. I wasn't going anywhere. I actually wondered what I would do once the Western Town was all built.

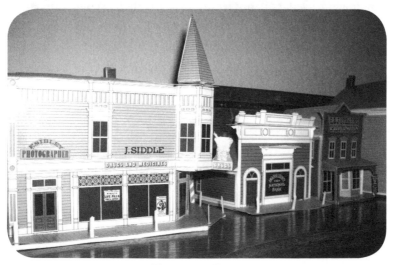

My Western Town.

A General Store sprung up out of nowhere, and a fancy hotel soon appeared next to it. My fingers hurt and leered at me, red and swollen, but I kept on going. That's all I knew how to do.

⌒

That same day, as I went to scratch my head, I noticed something peculiar. As I touched my scalp, it felt tender and sore, like a giant bruise. I pulled my hand away and along with it came many strands of hair. Uh-oh. I had asked Dr. Dan how long it would take until my hair would start falling out, but he had told me that it's different for everyone. Yikes, I was an early bird. Not quite believing it, I separated one tiny, microscopic hair from the rest and gently pulled it skyward. I was expecting a tug or some resistance, but received neither. Instead, I looked up. The hair completely detached from my head . . . I had not felt a single thing. I showed Mom, who shared in my deep fascination with my strange scalp. Just then, a lightbulb went on. I had an idea.

"Mom, I'm going to do a science experiment," I announced.

Her curiosity heightened, as I asked her to bring me the roll of duct tape from the garage. With the big gray roll in my hands, I stretched out a long piece and ripped it off. I pulled up my sweats and firmly pressed the tape onto my legs, which, as you can imagine, had not been shaven in quite awhile. In one fluid, sharp motion, I peeled it off, not feeling even the slightest ounce of pain.

Examining the tape, I observed the great amount of hair covering it. Yep, I was losing my hair alright . . . everywhere. Like Duct Tape Woman, I covered the rest of my legs with the silver, sticky stuff and repeated the process. Mom and I were cracking up; it beat shaving by a long shot. And, not only was I taking care of my overgrown leg hair, I was also taking care of my science for the day.

My hypothesis was that if my hair roots had died, then my hair could be plucked out with little or no pain. To confirm my surmise, I had Mom do the same on her legs. Um . . . not quite as successful and, I can imagine, a little bit painful. But Mom gave a sacrifice to science and also to my daily dose of laughter.

Although shocked to be losing my hair—the hair that everyone had always told me was so beautiful—I looked at it as a unique and different experience. The majority of human beings, especially teenagers, don't go through total hair loss. So, even though it was weird, shocking, and slightly disturbing, I "grew" to be fine with it.

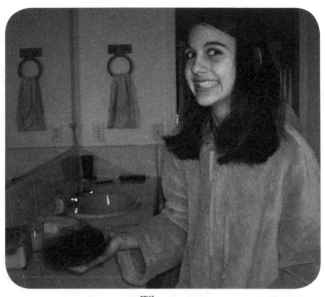

Whoa . . .

My pink beanie slid over my delicate head, probably yanking out even more precious hairs straight from the root. I slipped into a jacket. It was pleasant outside, but with a tiny winter chill still lingering in the pure Nipomo air. I was so excited about my little stroll the day before that I asked Mom if we could go on another one. Only this time, I wanted to walk down our street. I got the green light.

As I ventured outside for my second time, I filled my lungs with the crisp air. It refreshed me, not like the somewhat stuffy inside air. Everything was orange, as it always was that time of the day, and Mom took my arm and walked close to me. Descending the driveway, we made a sharp right when we reached the bottom. I was out, out of my comfort and safety zone, but it felt *good*. We inched along, and I smiled like I had won the World's Strongest Man Competition. The sensation of being outside fed my soul, and my tired, worn-out body got energy from somewhere . . . God's Earth, I guess.

"Now this is human," I thought.

I felt in my natural habitat outdoors. People are not meant to be indoors constantly, staying away from the beautiful world around us. We were created, like all animals, to roam the land. I pictured myself on *Animal Planet*, and smiled.

Raising my head, I peered up at the many, many trees situated in our neighbor's yards . . . they had grown. One thing that has always stayed with me is how bright and vivid the colors were that evening. The trees glowed with a green my eyes had not yet seen; the flowers sparkled in their colorful jackets; and the sky, an unbelievable and spectacular blue, gave way to the swirling sunset. Everything resembled a coloring book, neatly filled in with bright, fun crayons. It was beautiful, like nothing I had ever seen before. I examined Ambi and Rosalind's poppies. They've always had an immaculate and stunning yard. Just then, I realized how far I had walked and just how weak I was beginning to feel.

Mom must have read my mind because, right then, she asked, "You want to turn around?"

I nodded, slowly hanging a U-turn back toward our house. The long, straight road ahead of me displayed how far I had come and how far I would have to go to get back. The loose gravel on the edge of the street made a loud noise as my feet dragged through it. It became annoying, and I fought to pick my feet up higher.

All was quiet, except for the familiar sound of the neighborhood dogs barking as we walked past. We had been out for only five minutes, yet it seemed to me I had been out for an hour. This wasn't because each step required an extreme amount of energy, but because I treasured each movement and felt like all of time had frozen and ground to a halt.

It was all about me at that moment, and I imagined the trees, the grass, and the entire world watching me. Like a mother who witnesses her baby's first steps, God, His incredible world, and Mom witnessed mine. They were actually like "second" first steps, ones that probably meant just as much, if not more, than the very first. I felt like I was a baby again, getting fed, bathed, and comforted. After overcoming my primary resistance, I grew to accept it.

As Mom and I neared our home once again, something occurred to me. Not too many people experience babyhood twice, and no one, certainly, is able to remember it. I was blessed and cursed. I climbed up our driveway, my own personal "Stairway to Heaven." Milking my final steps, I was victorious, yet saddened. I had made a huge leap in my recovery, but now, I had to return to the bed that invisibly chained me down . . . my body told me to do so.

A smile broke out on my face like a pimple on a teenager. No more shots. Nurse Pam called, and she explained that my blood counts were good enough to discontinue the Neupogen shots for now. I still had the subsurface soreness in every bone, but was spared from the daily stick. So, that next morning, after I made it to the bottom of the little metal cup Mom piled my pills in, Mr. Anxiety didn't crawl out from his cave in the back of my head.

Although relieved that the pokes were temporarily discontinued, something much greater bothered me. It was dance . . . actually, the lack thereof. Having no idea when I would dance again gave me a feeling of loss of control. I could barely walk . . . how could I dance?

Classes were starting soon, and Youth Company auditions were right around the corner, mocking me. Youth Company is a group of the best dancers in the youth dance program. The previous fall had been my first time in Company, and I had looked forward to heightening my dance abilities, as well as performing as a Company member in the spring show for the very first time.

My dreams were crushed . . . there was no way I could maintain that schedule. Heck, I might not even be *able* to dance at all. My heart crumbled, like an eroding mountainside, and lay in a crumpled heap on the foot of the bed. My sobs were deep and pained, hard for even me to listen to. If there were only two things that I could have in this world, they would be my family and *dance*. I desired to be at the studio so badly that it hurt. That slipping feeling, that awful, helpless sensation of all that you have being taken from your very own hands came over me. I was powerless. I worried that the strength and skills I had developed in dance would quickly fade away, and I would be back at ground zero.

"It's not fair."

The words tumbled in my head like clean clothes in a dryer.

It sounds quite immature and stupid now, but I became very jealous of all the girls I knew from my classes. They got to dance. They got to have energy. They got to choose what they wanted to do.

They got to wake up every morning and *not* say, "I hope I feel okay today."

Suddenly, gratitude appeared, and all jealousy was strained from it. I set myself straight. I was *alive*; although my *pointe* shoes lay in the corner gathering a thin layer of dust . . . *I was alive.*

"Affliction comes to us all, not to make us sad, but sober; not to make us sorry, but to make us wise; not to make us despondent, but by its darkness to refresh us as the night refreshes the day; not to impoverish, but to enrich us." —Henry Ward Beecher

EIGHT

DAD NEARLY COLLAPSED, and his eyeballs bugged out from his head. I guess that was the first time he ever really noticed the progression, or shall I say regression, of my hair loss. What occurred was quite fascinating. I had expected for hair to fall out everywhere, leaving patches of hair and no hair until all was gone. But instead, my one-eighth-inch part grew wider and wider until a stripe of a little over an inch created almost a "freeway" on my head. Hmm . . . Route Baldo . . . kinda has a ring to it. Anyway, each attempt to brush my hair resulted in more lanes being added, my own personal "tax dollars" at work. I needed some cones to set out.

For some reason, the person most upset about me losing my hair was not Mom, not me, but Dad. Every time he would wander in from our spa, only to confront my widening strip, he took a harder hit. It was not sadness; it was shock . . . pure shock. I guess he didn't really enjoy seeing his daughter look like some creature out of *The Lord of the Rings*.

With my hair follicles disintegrating by the minute, Mom and I were bound for the wig shop. We had flung open the phone book to "W" and found a place fairly close that was open on Sundays. I wasn't freaking out about my fast approaching cue-ball appearance; rather, I saw it as an inevitable, odd, and twisted source of entertainment. I didn't feel like I *needed* a wig, or else I would have to crawl into a cave where I would remain for the duration of my treatment, IV pole and all.

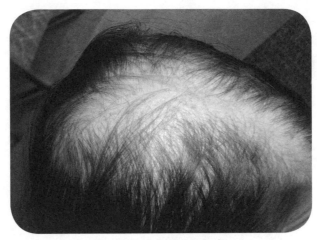

My *Lord of the Rings* look.

However, a dear friend of our family, who is lovingly dubbed Auntie Priscilla, insisted that she purchase the wig of my choice. It was so kind, and I began to realize, as we walked around the small shop, that there would be many times I would want to blend into the crowd. There was a difference between not caring about my baldness and just wanting to feel normal and not have the awkward stares.

The mass of manikin heads wore every shade and style of hair imaginable, but one wig immediately stood out, to both me and my mom. It looked very similar to my hair before I got sick: long and brown, but a tiny bit lighter in color. I had cut off that dark, long, lush hair of mine and sent it to Locks of Love the previous February, totally clueless of where I'd be in a year.

I joked with Dr. Dan, saying, "Maybe I'll get my own hair back!"

Funny how life can kill you with irony, huh? The déjà vu I felt when I put that wig on surprised me. I sat looking at my former self, and visions that came back made me happy, yet sad. The wig was truly beautiful, like a brunette Rapunzel. It was tucked into a small, golden box, neatly folded with a thin tissue paper layer. I was excited, my heartbeats like little hops on a pogo stick. Auntie Priscilla did such a wonderful thing for me that day, and I am so very grateful for it.

With my spirit flying high, but my body quickly tiring, we started for home. That was the first little outing I had, and it was incredible to feel a teeny sense of normality. But strangely, everything looked different as I peered out the passenger side window that day. It was not so much how things *looked* as how they *felt* . . . the energy emitted from them. It's so difficult to describe this sensation, but it was like nothing was familiar to me. Even though I had seen the McDonald's situated near our freeway on-ramp daily in the past, it felt alien to me. The visual memory was there, yet I took on the persona of an out-of-towner, a tourist.

My emotional connections and associations with things rotted away. Our library became just some library. I noticed how weird our bank looked, and even our street became just some neighborhood street. It's so very strange, and nearly impossible to describe. It's like taking a step back and disconnecting from everything you know. Suddenly, I saw things literally wider and broader. It was a change of perception.

With the car window separating me from the world, I felt like a foreigner from another planet, exploring in my silver spaceship. We arrived back home . . . just some house, and I crawled into my bed . . . just some bed.

☙

My brother hollered at the TV as the tiny men ran back and forth. I didn't really get football, still don't, and therefore couldn't get too jazzed over it. I, instead, sat sprawled on the floor, our low coffee table within an arm's reach. Running my fingers through my hair, I gathered more and more, a fairly large clump accumulating on the glass table. I wasn't trying to pull out my own hair; I was "de-shedding." It was starting to get *everywhere*, and I rivaled Larry, our dog, in hair distribution.

So, while my goal was to weed out the dead hairs, many healthy ones were extracted unintentionally. I continued the motion, and the pile grew larger. Suddenly, a big wad detached from the Mothership.

"Oh gyyyosh," I blurted.

It had become Mom's and my favorite line when anything unexpected happened. I added the clump to my collection. The mound resembled Chewbacca from *Star Wars*. All it needed were eyes, a mouth, and a nose. I literally heard Chewy's famous, lovable groan. Man, all of this shedding was a pain, and I already felt bad about all the vacuuming Mom would have to do. But, oddly enough, there was something soothing about sitting there yanking my hair out while watching sweaty dudes throw a ball around. The longer I sat there, the bigger Chewbacca became. By the fourth quarter, there lay more hair on the table than on my head. My family was shocked, as was I. My hair had essentially all fallen out in one epic day. And so, from that day on, January 12, 2008, has been remembered as *The Great Hair Fallout Day*.

The mirror was a visual aid in grasping the reality that I had just about as much hair as a naked mole rat. My male-pattern baldness was most prominent where my part once stood. From there on out, the forest became slightly thicker. The near crop circle on my head was disturbing, yet hilarious. The phases went from top to bottom, and looking into the future, I saw myself with almost a "curtain" of hair along the side of my head, but nothing on top. I laughed so hard that it hurt.

"Mom," I shouted, still in a slur of giggles, "I'm gonna look like Ben Franklin!"

We laughed until our bellies hurt, our eyes were watering, and we were nearly peeing in our pants. And then . . . we laughed some more.

Hmm. What to do with that giant pile of hair? Have some fun, of course. The irresistible mountain became a hat and sash for Carrie Bear. I must say, she looked rather stunning in it, like she was ready for fashion week in Paris. And then, after her photo shoot, Carrie's attire was saved in gallon-size Ziploc bags. Sometime forty years from now, I'll run across the hair I had when I was thirteen.

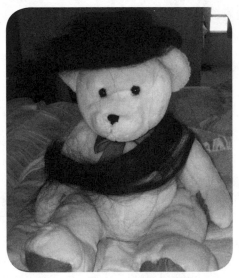

Carrie Bear on the Great Hair Fallout Day

I'll dig it up one day, when I'm old and brittle, and say, "This was Grandma's hair years and years ago, when I was your age. Now I'd like you to have it."

I can picture the "thanks, but no thanks" expression on my grandchild's face. Or maybe I'll begin to lose my hair when I'm old, and I'll have a stock to fill in the gaps.

As for the daily, individual hairs that leaped off my scalp, they went in the trash or out the car window. I remember asking Mom one day if it was considered littering. I added that I didn't believe so, because hair is natural. I thought birds could make very warm, beautiful nests out of it and that I must be doing them a huge favor. Here was my case: If you throw a booger out the window, is it considered littering? I concluded that I would not be getting fined any time soon.

The amazingly beautiful Santa Ynez Valley smiled back at me as it flew past. We were on our way to Santa Ynez Cottage Hospital for my very first post-chemo chest X-ray.

"2050 Viborg Road," I recited from memory, trying to assist Mom in locating it.

We found it tucked into a lot on a small side road . . . it was adorable. God shut the lights off and then back on as I got out of the car, probably way too fast. The sliding doors parted, and a quaint, old waiting room greeted us. After checking in at an interrogation-size room, I was called. By this time, I was a pro at the whole chest X-ray deal and could have done it with my eyes closed.

As I stood there, splattered against the target board like a swatted fly, I prayed for results. I prayed for death. Not of me, but *it*. After I had changed back into my own clothes, I emerged from the tiny curtain-closed room.

"Can we see them?" I heard Mom ask the technician.

"Sure," he replied, tilting the computer screen toward us.

Whoa, it was my chest. White areas illustrated bones, organs, and tissues. I saw a lot of it. My invasive blob was quite apparent, and I silently snarled at it. It didn't answer back. It was so weird looking at me but being myself all at the same moment. It was confusing to my mind, this being the first personal X-ray it had seen.

"Wow! That used to be all white there," Mom observed, pointing to a dark black area.

I held my breath. I was overjoyed. My giant mass had responded rapidly to the chemo—it was shrinking.

Gleaming smiles broke out on our faces, and I knew that we were thinking the exact same thing . . . "*Thank you, God.*"

And that is just about all we said as we prayed and rejoiced driving back through the never-ending vineyards. The afternoon light rested upon their leafy rows, matching the way I felt inside—beautiful.

❦

Dr. Dan seemed very pleased with my tumor's response, or he would not have agreed to the port implant. We would venture to Cottage Hospital that night and sleep over at the Best Western across the street. Early the next morning, I would have my port inserted, and shortly thereafter, begin my second round of chemotherapy.

I vividly remember the evening drive down to Santa Barbara. Before leaving home, I had shoved stuffed animals, pillows, and blankets into the car. I had wolfed down a plate full of mac 'n cheese like I would never eat again. Then, I had grabbed a pile of cookies for the trek.

Listening to the radio, my spirits were unusually high for, once again, entering the chemo war zone. I remember dancing to the different songs that came on. It was the most fun I had had in a long while. My anxiety was minimal because I was more experienced and prepared this time. Still, that wouldn't make anything easier.

❦

I squeezed into the tightly tucked hotel sheets and flipped on the TV. The bed constricted me, and I kicked to loosen things up a bit. It was a cute room, one with high ceilings and big mirrors. The Teddy Bear Cancer Foundation paid for it, a small act of kindness that meant so much more than it seemed. My gratitude was interrupted by *American Idol* coming on. For a few years now, Mom and I have been parked together in front of the TV virtually every Tuesday night. It isn't because we have an obsession with the show; rather, it serves as a time to be with one another.

I grinned, my head popping out of my own personal queen size bed. A lot may have been taken from me, but I still had my Tuesday nights with Mom. It was the very first episode of the *American Idol* season, and they were auditioning in Philadelphia. We watched and listened as they briefly told of the city's history.

Suddenly, someone familiar popped up on the screen. It was Ben. Ben Franklin. Mom and I lost it, completely lost it. Our laughter could probably be heard throughout the entire hotel. We laughed so hard, one of the most gut-wrenching laughs I have ever experienced. The only thing that made me stop was my light head and difficulty breathing . . . it was awesome.

The morning came too soon, and the foggy, cold weather bid us good day. A slight uncertainty bubbled inside of me, but other than that, I was ready. I had gotten used to surrendering my body. Totally disconnecting from it, I was able to lessen my emotional pain. I truly thought of myself in two parts: my body and my spirit. As far as I was concerned, crud could mess with my body, but *nothing* could take over and control my spirit. That was comforting to me, knowing that whatever physical torment I had to go through, it was just my body and not my soul. Like an old boyfriend, I was *so* over my body.

Pre-op questions began.

"What is your name? When's your birthday? How old are you? What are you here for?"

The obvious, yet necessary, questions went on and on as the nurses began to hook me up, as though they were jumping a car.

I knew that their intentions were safety, but I thought, "Why are you asking me? You're the one with my chart!"

For reasons unknown to me, I do not remember this day very well. Who knows, maybe I decided right there on that stretcher that I would forget the whole ordeal. My parents looked down at me, in fact everyone did . . . it felt weird. The only thing I recall is Dr. Keshen and the nurses laughing as I drifted off. I must have said something funny.

The next memory is pain. I felt it even before I opened my eyes. When I did open them, I carefully lifted my gown to examine Dr. Keshen's work. I saw one incision, no wait, two, and a small lump that, ironically, resembled a tumor. I looked up and saw Dr. Willsey entering. He reassured me by confirming that the procedure had gone well, despite there having been one tiny obstacle. They had originally planned to make an incision on the left, but something that had to do with my PICC line, which was on the left, prevented them from doing so. Now, I had a cut on the right, a cut on the left, *and* a slice in the middle. Looking at it made it hurt more.

I was taken back to the Peds octopus room, called this because of the large picture of the eight-legged animal mounted on the wall opposite my bed. Every ocean-inspired room displayed a different sea creature. Quite fittingly, I received the octopus. I still had my extra limb, my PICC line, and I knew just how that octopus felt. They couldn't remove it during my surgery because they were using it to administer my anaesthesia. They wanted it to be free for the off chance of me needing medication immediately.

So, there I was, a tube coming out of my arm and a port in my chest, receiving fluids and prepping for chemo. And that's not even counting my blood pressure cuff, blood oxygen reader, and the digital thermometer sitting on the table nearby, ready to take my temperature at any moment.

Whatever they gave me for pain during the port implantation began to wear off, and I was left in sheer misery. It was unbelievable, and practically unbearable. Moving was impossible. Suddenly realizing how uncomfortable I had become, lying in the same position, I attempted a move. Yikes. Nope, definitely wasn't gonna happen.

As time passed, it began to hurt with each breath. The incision was slightly to the left of the center of my chest, and it stretched back and forth as I sucked in and blew out. I couldn't take it any longer; it was just too painful. I gathered all of the strength I had and asked for something, anything, to numb me. They did the whole "pain scale" thing, "1" being nothing and "10" being highly unbearable. I think I chose about a nine, and I usually underestimate the severity of my discomfort.

My nurse returned with morphine, the king of all painkillers. I'm not exactly sure why, but it was kind of scary as she added it to the fluids draining into me. Maybe it was the fact that I *did* need such a potent painkiller, which meant that my suffering was pretty serious and pretty extreme. Or maybe it was just the name "morphine," another medically related word that sounds much more frightening than it actually is. Never in my life would I have imagined that I would be lying in the hospital, getting pounded with morphine, at age thirteen.

With my eyes drooping, I began to be able to relax slightly. The pain was still there, but my extreme drowsiness blurred it. I could breathe easier, but was careful not to inhale too deeply for fear that the sharp, shooting pain radiating from my incision and shaking my fragile nervous system would return. I felt so drugged-out, yet relieved, all at the same moment. In a sick, twisted way, I enjoyed my dazed mind and numbed state.

Around this time, I was visited by family friends we've known forever. We love them so greatly . . . it's a beautiful friendship. They are always there for us, and we are always there for them. Our mutual support for each other keeps bringing us closer and closer to each other's hearts.

Vicki and John, who we call "JY," drove north to Cottage Hospital from their Los Angeles home to bring me hugs, smiles, love, and encouragement. JY, one of the funniest guys walking the Earth, brought along his jokes, his loud, booming voice, and his complete obliviousness to all embarrassment. When I saw his huge bobble head pop in the door, with his ear-to-ear grin, I forgot about every pain, every discomfort, and every *itch*. And Vicki; her sweet, glowing face brings peace to the most stressful situations. Between the two of them and Mom and Dad, it was a serene, tranquil Garden of Eden . . . or the closest thing to it at least.

Like Superman, JY flew in to save me from reaching the point of complete insanity. Donning a cut, tan plastic glove on his head, he exploded into my room. After the barrels of laughter he received faded, he explained to me the intentions he had. He wanted to make me feel less alone, with virtually only a few strands of hair still clinging to my head. So somewhere between me and JY with his bald cap, there was a click . . . a bond. Leave it to JY to be comforting and hysterical all at the same moment. I tell you, you can laugh one second and cry the next with that guy . . . I love him to death.

Even though there were strange looks from the medical staff, he kept the jokes flying. They dove right in, whipped out their feathers, and tickled my heart. JY and Vicki, as well as the morphine, kept me in a happy place despite my plight. I truly believe that the laughter and love surpassed the morphine in relieving my pain.

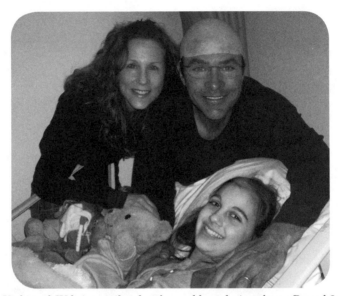

Vicki and JY bring smiles, laughs, and love during chemo Round 2.

Uncertainty raced through my body as I heard the "snap, snap" of gloves slipping over Dr. Dan's skilled hands. Positioning himself beside my bed, he slowly began stripping off the tape that kept my PICC line in place.

I almost yelled, "No, wait! I want anaesthesia!" but he told me it was painless, and I wouldn't feel any discomfort.

As he peeled off the tape, I grimaced as the few remaining hairs I had were ripped out by their roots. I turned my head, staring at the blank wall, as tension invaded me. Dr. Dan began. I experienced no pain, but it kind of . . . well, tickled. Deep inside my vein, I could feel something brushing and rubbing as it traveled through. The subsurface sensation started from my chest and traveled around the bend of my shoulder before continuing down my arm. The hole in my arm, through which it escaped, also tickled with a strange feeling. It resembled the feeling of when you slurp spaghetti, only coming out instead. It was *weird*—like something out of a horror/sci-fi movie. I imagine that it looked even weirder than it felt.

Just then, the sensation ended, and looking back to Dr. Dan, I saw a long, white tube wound up like a snake in his hand. Examining the quarter, or so, inch hole in my arm, I half expected blood to come spewing out everywhere, erupting like Mt. St. Helens. But it was just *there*, and it was creepy.

Eyeing the occupants of my bed, I smiled as Danny, my stuffed dog, came into view. Jaynie and I had played with him pre-op, and he was now fully dressed in bright blue, non-latex-smelling apparel. He looked adorable. There had been quite a bit of waiting before my surgery that morning, like there always seemed to be before an operation. What do you suppose the medical staff is doing during that time? Cleaning up from the last one or something? Or maybe they're down at the coffee shop, shooting the breeze. Who knows?

Anyway, during that awkward time, Jaynie kept me busy, leaving not a moment for me to ponder my approaching surgery. Discreetly "borrowing" scrubs and items from the hospital, we dressed up Danny, as well as Antonio, my gorilla, before setting them up for a photo shoot. When I was first called into Peds, a somber feeling had come over me. Anxious waiting had been turned into fun that I wished would never end.

So, as I reposed, observing Jaynie's and my handiwork, I pictured what it would be like to play with Jaynie in the hospital *all day long* . . . without any test, chemo, or misery. It would be heaven.

The saying "All good things must come to an end" is so very true.

It seems that a high is followed by a low, and a low is followed by a high. That's how I feel my life has been, and although exhausting, the bad times make me appreciate the good times, and the good times . . . well . . . they just *rock*.

With my nausea better controlled this round, I didn't have nearly as rough a time as the first. However, each round proved to have its own unique challenges, and for Round 2, it was pain. Even with the morphine, I can still remember my ultimate inability to move, even the slightest inch. I recall turning my head, the only part of my body I could move with only minimal discomfort. I stared at my pink bucket on the bedside table, and it took me a moment to process what had been drawn on its rosy face.

With many black Sharpie drawn flowers, it read, "Barf Bucket," in huge, looping letters.

Great. Thanks. Appreciate it. Don't get me wrong, it was sweet and all . . . just minus the whole "barf" part. Part of me enjoyed that the nurses didn't beat around the bush, but got straight to the point. That's what it was, a puke bucket. It wasn't a toy boat, a giant cereal bowl, or a tub used by a busboy to clear tables. You threw up in it . . . period. And as the bright afternoon transformed into black-bearded night, I was happy to discover that I only needed that stupid, beautiful, horrible, thoughtful, blushing bucket two times.

⤳

I can evoke exactly how I felt as I sat slouched over, like the Hunchback, in the hospital bathroom: burning up in a fire of misery. Mom and I were jammed into the tiny area, and all was deathly quiet, except for the whoosh-whoosh of my IV pump, Ricco. I was done, but could not summon up the amazing degree of strength it would take to rise, and so, I just waited, for what . . . I don't know. In those moments, I not only *felt* like I was dying, I realized that I practically *was* dying. Nothing is worse than noticing how sick you are. To make it through a serious and traumatic medical event, you have to be somewhat in denial about your condition.

My head hung, with nothing but my rubbery neck keeping it off the floor. I eyed the bright red emergency string attached to the dimly lit wall and prayed I would never have to use it. I remained strong . . . I was doing it. And then, suddenly, my view rotated, and I found myself in a staring contest with Ricco. After many silent moments faded away, I displayed my disapproval of my new, conjoined twin.

Shaking my head, I wriggled my nose, sarcastically, at "him," as if to say, "I hate you!"

Mom, who stood like the ref of our stare-down, chuckled. She rubbed her face and confessed, "I needed that."

Even though my nausea and stomach pains ebbed in severity from the first round, the night was a battle, a struggle. I kept pushing to withstand my pain, my queasiness, and, well . . . everything. It's so scary when you have to put all that you've got into fighting and have to concentrate on being so strong, especially emotionally and spiritually. I know for a fact that at any point in my treatment, I could have literally chosen to die. At any moment, I had the power to decide if I wanted to live, or if I desired to die. Other people could save me physically from dying, but as far as I was concerned, if I gave up spiritually, it was the end.

Our minds are such complex devices and our spirits such intricate webs. Our thoughts and feelings influence our bodies so greatly that when we lose our will and strength mentally, we also lose it physically.

I told Mom, only a short time into treatment, "Cancer is 20 percent physical, 80 percent mental."

Behind the chemo-curtain of my newly opened eyes, I saw my grandparents. I don't recall what time it was, because my biological clock was literally smashed to pieces. The concept of day and night for me was not significant. Their expressions morphed dramatically when their minds processed what they were viewing. I could tell it was hard for them, and I felt bad. I hate making things hard for people. But I had no control over my shocking and downright frightening appearance. I actually remember trying to look as well as possible for my visitors.

The absolute last thing I wanted was for someone to come in teary-eyed, their bottom lip in a quivering, pouting position, and say, "Aw, you poor thing."

I couldn't handle that. So I did a good job of faking my well-being, and Gramma and Poppy did a good job of hiding their awe. A strange atmosphere surrounds hospital visits. A note of denial and disbelief is certain to be sensed, and the odd location kind of throws everyone off. Although they were a little awkward and slightly embarrassing for me, visits always gave me a mental and spiritual escape from my physical chains. I constantly felt like I was in another world, and seeing friends and family reminded me that I was still here on Earth. It snapped me back to reality.

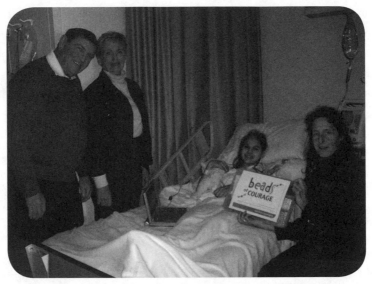

Distraction and love from Poppy, Gramma, and Jaynie.

My illness also made it possible for me to meet wonderful people I would not have had the honor of knowing otherwise. Casey Roberts is a beautiful example of a friend and human being. I cannot imagine *not* having met him because his humor, love, encouragement, and spirituality poured into my soul, giving me exactly what I needed to recover.

A high school classmate of Mom's, Casey lives in Santa Barbara. Every round, without fail, his calming demeanor filled my hospital room. His heart is so close to the Lord that you can feel God's holy presence shining through him, making his brown eyes twinkle behind his small, round glasses. He had stopped by my first round, but I only vaguely remember the blur of a stranger as I faded in and out of sleep. Mom had described him to me, but now I finally got to meet him.

The instant he walked in, even before he said a single word, he captured my heart. He looked at me as if I was his own daughter, and in my eyes, he was a father figure. The pureness of his heart and his words were the crisp, clear, iridescent waters that flowed through him. Peering up at him while snuggled deep in the covers of my creaking bed, I studied his ways. He is a supreme example of a humble and modest person, and the cream of the human race crop.

Petting his furry, black ears, I admired his innocence and unconditional love. Sammy, the therapy dog, lay sprawled on my bed, his thick tail thumping against the sheets. His calming aura soothed me, and I began to talk about the similarities between Sammy and our Labrador, Larry. They were very much alike, from their slightly doofy expressions, to their clumsiness that makes them adorable. The only difference, I said, was that Larry could not come up on the bed at home. Jaynie, who stood nearby, stepped forward, her mouth agape and her jaw hanging loose.

"What? Why not?" she asked, her face twisted into a shape I had never witnessed before.

"Well," I began, "my dad won't let him."

The Mama Bear in Jaynie came out, and I could see in her eyes that, within a matter of days, Larry would be crashed out in bed with me. Expressing my extreme doubt that my dad would ever allow it, I watched Jaynie form huge, clear letters with a bright blue marker on a large sheet of ivory-white paper. Like *Wheel of Fortune*, she flipped it around, showcasing her artistry. I chuckled.

It read, "I am good therapy (Woof!)."

She placed it next to Sammy and declared the kick start of the Let-Larry-on-the-Bed Campaign. I bet you are wondering who won . . . who do you think?!

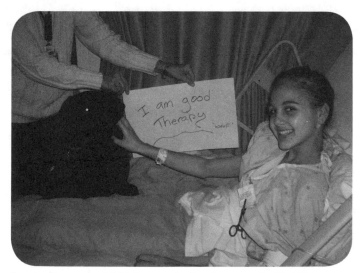

Jaynie, Sammy, and I kick-start the Let-Larry-on-the-Bed Campaign.

Nurse Cyndi's cheeks reddened as her eyes became two tiny, squinted lines. The laugh that escaped her was a result of my story. I had told her about me being Ben Franklin.

Once she gathered herself, she cackled, "That is so cute! You're my little Ben."

As she exited my room to get a fresh, spanking new bag of chemo, she instructed, "Now you have to think of a name for me."

I pondered the proper nickname. She arrived in her protective garb, the orange bag floating in her hand.

As if executing it, she hung the bag on my IV pole and asked, "Have you thought of a name for me yet?"

I paused, but only for a moment, before I blurted, "You're the Blue Chemo Fairy."

Her contagious giggle broke out and transformed into a high-pitched eruption of laughter.

When I told her, "And you bring chemo-fairy-pee," my creative, childlike mind sucked every fluid ounce of innocence from my bones and opened the flood gates.

I envisioned Cyndi, with wings and a small wand, hovering over the children with her magic chemo-fairy-pee, her bright blue robe sparkling in the light. Imagination is endless, and for that next bag of chemotherapy, all I thought about was my Blue Chemo Fairy, Cyndi. My vision came alive as the bright markers Jaynie had delivered to me re-created a 2-D picture of Nurse Cyndi, the Blue Chemo Fairy. Using every speck of concentration I could muster up, I paid close attention to capture the special essence she possessed. I scrupulously added the red detail to her Puma sneakers, and when the drawing was complete, I was proud. Anxiously awaiting the picture presentation for Nurse Cyndi, I became excited and restless. I knew that she would love it, and I loved doing something for her . . . she was, after all, helping save my life.

I know, I know, you're probably thinking, "A picture for your *life*?!"

Yep, a picture.

What else could I do?

Certainly, I wasn't going to lie there all day, repeating, "Thank you, thank you, thank you, thank you," until my face turned blue.

Plus, when you're younger like that, especially a cancer kid, you can draw a line on a piece of paper, give it to someone with a smile, and I can guarantee they'll respond, "Aw! I love it."

So when I held up that Blue Chemo Fairy, almost as if she were flying in mid-air, I saw Nurse Cyndi's broad smile. That's all I needed, that one look. My heart dropped, a happy drop, a grateful drop, a proud drop. I think it touched her. It's all a cycle, I tell you. She taped it up on her locker, probably after she was done parading it around the nurse's station. I can bet it's still there now, over a year later, the tape slightly peeling, the colors slightly faded, but my love still shining through.

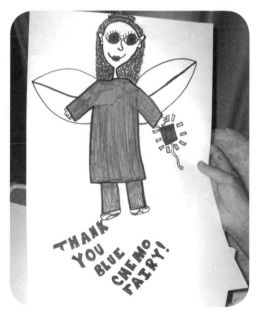

Nurse Cyndi, the Blue Chemo Fairy.

"Everybody can be great because everybody can serve . . .
you only need a heart full of grace. A soul generated by love."
—Martin Luther King Jr.

NINE

MY PINK BUCKET stood nearby in the backseat of the car, in case the winding roads should trigger an onslaught of nausea. I really hoped they wouldn't. We were on our way home after War 2, oh . . . I mean Round 2. Each sweeping corner I'd brace to fight my queasiness, and it became highly exhausting. Reaching a fairly straight stretch of road, I did exactly what I did my first round: I thought about how much I'd done, and how much was left. Always at that little valley, just before the turnoff for Nojoqui Falls and The Blueberry Farm, I reassured myself.

"I've already done *two*," I told myself, while my lips remained idle.

"Two rounds. I'm *halfway* there . . . halfway," I asserted. "Only two more, two more . . . I can do it . . . two more."

However, my "two more" was measured by *rounds* of chemo. This was not including post-chemo radiation, or recovery. But all that was too overwhelming to even let enter my mind. It was a "cross-that-bridge-when-you-come-to-it" sort of thing. So I focused on the smaller goals. Actually, with cancer, the end of each day is a goal, and waking up in the morning is a victory. You literally take it, not day by day, but minute by minute, second by second. All time is slowed to a ridiculous pace, and it gives you a new insight into life and your values. It gives you way too much time to think, which can be good and it can be bad. You realize how much people get caught up in everyday life, and how they lose sight of what really matters.

I think it's strange what people choose to do with their lives. A person who is healthy, smart, and strong will go sit behind a desk, sipping their coffee and shuffling papers from nine to five. Then they will sit in traffic, get home, and pretty much go to bed. To me, that is sad . . . pitiful.

I would like to ask that person, "Are you happy every day?"

I can almost guarantee the answer would be, "No."

So many of us lead bland, tasteless, hum-drum lives, with our potential lying lifeless, dusty, and cobweb-ridden in the corner. I guess that when you're severely sick and know it, and feel it *every second*, you become determined to make every second count for the rest of your life.

Yearning for my bed, I buried my head in my pillow, the seat belt the only thing keeping me vertical. I knew that nothing would stop me once I was well, healed. I was so sure that I was going to make something of my life, and celebrate it every day until I die.

☞

"I feel like a walking pharmacy," I told Mom as a tray appeared on my lap, with more pills than breakfast.

In reply, I got a chuckle filled with empathy. The day proved to be a typical one. My port hurt, my face remained jammed in my pillow for the duration of the day, and the prednisone that became momentarily lodged in the back of my throat made for a permanent bitter taste, which made me even more nauseous than I already was. But through all of this, gratefulness flickered in my heart. The first round had shown me just how close to dying I could come, so I was thankful for any improvement, no matter how small.

Like a giant callous, I was starting to build up my ability to cope with feeling ill. I focused on what was going right and what made me happy. Still, I'm far from perfect, and at times, I realized just how miserable I was. Disgusted with myself for crying, I would force myself to stop, and then, once again, I would be as cool as a cucumber, as if not a tear had been shed. That's how it's always been for me: either tranquil, calm seas or total breakdown, a tsunami. I have no in between.

☞

Later that same evening, after examining the loose hair when I lifted my head off the pillow, I made the choice. With Mom on one side and Nicholas on the other, we crawled down the hallway, as if preparing for launch. My hand grasped the metal hair buzzer on our bathroom counter. I was ready. With a "click," I fired it up . . . all eyes watched my steady hand. As though using my own personal, mini-lawn mower, I executed a perfectly straight line from the center of my forehead to the crown of my head.

I paused. It was an epic moment, and I knew it . . . everyone did. The now free hair floated elegantly down to the waiting floor as I began to form a parallel row. Feeling the cool air on my bare head, I giggled. It was something virtually no one experiences, let alone a thirteen-year-old girl.

I followed the contour of my head. I had never really known what shape it was. The tiny, delicate hairs slid down the back of my shirt, making me itchy. Carefully, I formed a giant circle on the top of my head, trying hard to make it as even as possible. The circle grew larger, just as a crop circle mysteriously forms in cornfields at 3:00 a.m.

Suddenly, I stopped and stared at the stranger reflected back at me. I had purposely ceased midway to, truly, be the one I resembled. I *was* Ben Franklin. With only straggly hair running around the majority of my head's circumference, I depicted the founding father perfectly! Laughter erupted, and I found a chuckle that squeezed shock, excitement, embarrassment, and joy right out of me.

After a Kodak moment with Nicholas, "Ben," and Ben on a one-hundred-dollar bill, I retrieved the hair buzzer once again. I couldn't stay Little Ben forever. Within moments, I was clean shaven, the floor littered with a thin layer of hair. It was like someone had "cut and pasted" my hair off of my head and onto the floor. It was there, and then it was gone. I couldn't stop rubbing my head, the tiny remaining stubs tickling my fingers, and my soft touch creating a unique sensation on my sensitive skin.

Looking up, my eyes met my dad's . . . he had just come in from our spa, and his jaw hung open. He was completely in awe . . . he looked at the bathroom like it was a war zone.

It was entirely silent, and I gave him a smile that read, "Heeeeyyyyy! What's up?"

Mortification permeated his stunned face and, at last, he choked out, "I can't believe it."

He noticed the slew of hair littering the off-white linoleum floor and cringed, "I—I don't know what to say."

When I fell into bed and put my head onto my hair-covered pillow, it was like a newly exposed bowling ball dropping into a sandbox.

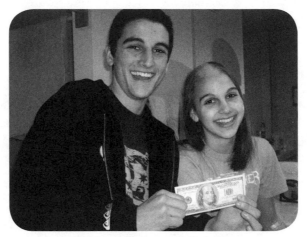

Nicholas, real Ben, and Little Ben.

The front door squeaked open the next morning, and with its usual loud, wooden clunk, it closed.

"Click, click, click!"

The incoming person locked it tightly behind them. Dean, who had slept at a friend's house the night before, appeared around the corner, my bald head instantly mesmerizing him.

"Mushy!" he yelled as he rushed toward me.

As he stroked my head like a dog, I felt a special connection with him, like big brother was there so nothing bad would, or could, possibly happen. It was a cold morning, and Dean was wearing his thick, dark brown visor beanie. Unexpectedly, he removed it and placed it on my head. It was a gesture of love I will never forget, with his smile even warmer than the beanie.

These are the moments that I have treasured. People wonder, how can you possibly "treasure" *cancer*?! It's the moments of nothing but pure love and joy that make the horrible times crumble . . . it's then.

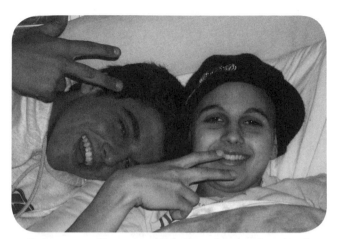

Peace out . . . Dean warming both my heart and my head.

I smothered EMLA cream onto the site of my port. I have to admit, I was nervous and brimming with anxiety. The EMLA cream numbed it up pretty well, but I was still apprehensive about Amalia coming to draw labs. Only under sedation had my port been "accessed," or poked. Now, I would have to remain calm as a needle sped toward my chest, hopefully landing in the exact spot, and at the exact angle, to hit the inch-wide margin that left little room for error.

I heard a car door . . . crud. I wanted to remain snuggled under my blue, angel-soft blanket watching *Match Game* so badly, but I knew that there was no avoiding it. I felt like I had been put into a washing machine, whirling around with an amazing amount of force. Then, the cycle stopped, and although still disoriented and confused, I momentarily got a taste of serenity. Suddenly, a new cycle would begin, and I was violently tossed around once again. Daily life was a Maytag. My only problem was . . . it had endless cycles.

The "drain" cycle fired up, but instead of removing water, the incentive was sucking up blood. Amalia wore her usual, business-like face as she sterilized just about everything she could sterilize. That included me, who lay on the edge of the bed with my shirt pulled up almost to my ears. It wasn't the most pleasant experience, having my entire chest scrubbed to a state of perfection—it actually kind of hurt.

I wanted to rub the irritated skin but received a "No! No! No! Don't touch it," just centimeters away from doing so.

"Wow. It's way down there!"

Yep. Most ports are in the upper chest, in the nearby neck area, but Dr. Keshen had placed mine lower so it wouldn't show when I wore my dance costumes. I thought it was extremely sweet and thoughtful of him. But as Amalia began to manipulate it, moving it the way she desired for better access, I couldn't look. It hurt. It was creepy. It was weird.

Sighing, I wrenched my head to look out the window. It was one of those helpless sighs, the big, drawn-out kind. Amalia was robotic—preparing vials, needles, tubes, gauze pads, you name it—which didn't settle my uprising anxiety. Amalia's glove-covered hand dove in like a pelican, and she began the search for my port. My face twisted and cringed as she pushed and, finally, stuck the needle in my port.

I find it quite hysterical, now, that I actually became used to it. That became the norm for me, having someone poke and prod for it before flying in with the all-important stick. A needle in your chest is kind of strange, as I have only recently discovered. And boy, that little devil caused more pain for me psychologically than anything else. I felt pressure, almost as if my chest was going to collapse in on me, and only a small prick as it slid into my port. Once in, I consciously and blatantly avoided having it even in my peripheral vision.

I remember thinking, "Hmm . . . there's a needle in my chest. Not exactly something you do every day . . . hmm, interesting."

It's amazing how your body not only defends you physically, but your mind defends you psychologically.

The sharp, pacifier-shaped needle sat lodged in my left breast, for gosh sake, and all I could do to react was, "Hmm . . . interesting."

☙

The morning prednisone was taking effect. "Mushy having a moooooooood swiiiiiiiing!" I yelled, feeling irritable.

It had become my new prednisone catch line, said sarcastically as well as truthfully. I don't like being crabby, and it is rough when you can't exactly help it.

So, I had to be content with saying, "Sorry, I'm feeling crabby," at multiple times throughout the day.

Knitting helped with keeping my snapping to a minimum. The vigorous clicking of the needles exhausted some of the day's frustrations. I am one who believes in productive release of emotions. Hats and scarves appeared as my fragile mind was numbed by the repetitive, monotonous motion. This was certainly much better than just lying there in my own pile of pooh.

Yet, sometimes, anything and everything that I did became frustrating, like a burr under my already irritated saddle. My tolerance for anything remotely pestering was wearing as thin as a blade of grass, and occasionally, even a task as simple as knitting morphed into an unbelievable struggle.

I recall trying to knit a hat once, with multiple balls of flashy yarn strung all across the bed. Focusing and clicking away for hours, I finally completed it. I noticed then that it was *tiny*, and I mean *teeny tiny*. Grabbing my stuffed polar bear, Poley, I jammed it on his head . . . oh well. The next item was just as much of a failure. It could barely be called a hat, and it had a big hole in the top, with a fairly large flap in the back.

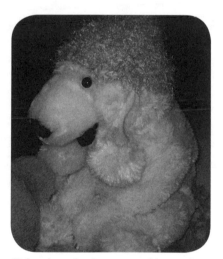

Poley the polar bear wears his new hat.

Disgusted with my waste of yarn and time, I threw it to the side. Truly believing that the third time would, in fact, be the charm, I was bitterly disappointed as my hard work turned into a "pancake hat," completely flat. Mom said it would make a beautiful coaster, but I could only force out a miserable chuckle. It was one that started out normal but, about halfway through, got infused with a whiny tone. So eventually, I gave up entirely on Project Hat and just stuck to scarves.

The following day, January 22, was an extremely difficult one. On top of my inhumane physical symptoms, my heart crumbled like a mountainside within me. It was the first day of dance of the new semester . . . and I wasn't able to go. I believe that this day I cried more than I remained dry-eyed, with a lump in my throat the size of a tennis ball.

I remember moaning, "The other girls get to go. Why can't I go to dance?"

Mom, who picked up my shattered soul off the fading carpet, used tender, yet truthful, words to soothe me.

"Because you have a very important job to do right now."

Frustration flew out of me.

"But they don't even have to think about not being well enough to go! They can just say, 'I'm gonna dance today.' It's not fair."

"I know, I know."

She tried her best to console me as her gentle hand rubbed my back. A blubbering mess, I was entirely overwhelmed with my unfortunate plight. How is it that some girls, who maybe didn't even appreciate being able to dance, get to dance, and the girl whose *soul needs* to dance is trapped within a body that won't let her?

I was still naive about this whole matter at the time, but I would soon discover the precious gift I received from having to sit on the sidelines while everyone else basked in the fun. I cried so hard that it hurt, and I felt like my spirit was being melted in acid. I couldn't take it. Cancer had now taken away my love, my joy . . . and I was pissed. If I didn't have dance, what did life matter? The wave of difficult days continued, and I was being forcefully dragged down by the weariness of long-term illness.

I apparently yelled—half-joking, half-serious—to Mom, "If I sit around any longer, I'm gonna need Tylenol for my @$$!"

Yep, I sure was getting sick of being sick, and that made for sick × sick. Sick squared. And sick times anything equals even bigger problems.

"Ballet is a dance executed by the human soul."
—Alexander Pushkin

TEN

I HUMMED CONTENTEDLY as we zoomed down the 101 Freeway, with Cottage Hospital as our destination. It was time for the last day of chemo—Round 2—at the clinic. Although my body was about to be injected with poison once again, it felt wonderful to go somewhere. That bed in the living room, the one I won't dare lie down on anymore, was getting as old as the TV game show reruns at 10:00 a.m. on weekdays. I appreciated seeing the clouds and sky, the rolling hills, and the yellow and purple wildflowers that had begun to sprout up in droves.

Nature made me happy, and fresh air revived my chemical-ridden body. Admiring the lovely, sunny, Santa Barbara day, I unsteadily entered the sliding doors of the hospital. I was walking. When offered a wheelchair by Mom, I firmly declined. I was determined to get up to the clinic myself this time. Why? Because I could. As I strolled up to the check-in window at the clinic, I was positive that I would never again take walking for granted.

Nurse Pam smiled down at me, "Yeah, you look much perkier this time around."

It was true, and all of the staff at the clinic was in accord. But my gut feeling told me that, within a few hours, the chemo would be fully circulating, causing trauma to my small, unsuspecting body. My nerves tensed up, like something had pulled a drawstring within me. I watched as the worst of them all, the king of the chemos, was prepped beside me. It was Vincristine, the one I hated most.

Injected through a tiny syringe, I could tell that it was strong . . . very strong, because of its small, concentrated dose. And although it was little, it sure did spin me for a loop. The side effects that Vincristine tortured me with were some of the most severe of all five of the drugs. Jaw pain was a big one. You may be thinking that a little bit of a sore jaw is nothing, but this kind of pain was different. It was quick, sharp, and shooting, yet burning and constant. My head always felt like mush after Vincristine, like it was tightly clamped in a vice and then suddenly released.

Also, the harmless-looking fluid caused "reversible nerve problems," which created very distinct and unique tingling in my hands and feet. It made me feel like I had been in a massage chair for eight hours—numb beyond numb all over, and in places where one does not wish to be numb.

So, as the liquid slowly drained into me, I sighed, waiting for the onset of unpleasant symptoms. A giant "thunderstorm" was in the distance. I knew it was only a matter of time before I was in the eye of the storm.

More sarcastic than truthful, I joked, "Thanks for the chemo!" as I hopped down off of the table and waved.

Exiting through the tall doorway, I heard chuckles behind me. They continued echoing down the long hallway . . . I don't think that they had ever heard anything like that from one of their "kids."

⌒

I soon realized that the "thunderstorm" in the distance was actually a hurricane, a tornado, a monsoon. Changing dramatically from hot to cold, I fought a kind of chills that I had never experienced before. The tiny pins and needles that pricked my body were unusually severe. Our thermometer told us that I had a fever, and I experienced a pounding headache in addition. Mom looked at information from Dr. Dan. We were to call if my fever reached 101.5 degrees, and it hovered right below.

I wondered why I was feeling differently and became scared that I was hit with some kind of a reaction or something. The most terrifying thing was my heart. Like *The Little Engine That Could*, it pumped so hard, and so fast, that I feared it might stop. All of these issues, I thought, were just what I had to deal with, they were part of treatment.

I vividly remember a big box sitting only a foot or so away from me on the bed. It had come in the mail, and it sat there beside a pair of scissors, begging to be opened. Staring at it, I desired so much to rip it open, like on Christmas Day, but when I went to move . . . oh . . . nope. It was not going to happen. Wishing I had X-ray vision—even better, present-opening vision—I finally gripped the fact that I was entirely immobile, completely idle.

The numbers on the clock faded from one to another; I only felt worse. Mom assisted me in finally opening up the box. A rainbow-colored blanket jumped out, with hugs and kisses from our friend Cecile. It went from box to Melinda, me wrapping it around my frigid, yet burning, body as if it were a boa constrictor. I remember the smell of that blanket. It was unique. I concluded that it must be what her house smelled like, although the chemo probably masked the true scent. And so I snuggled, looking like Joseph in his Technicolor Dreamcoat, waiting patiently for my wave of torture to be over.

Unfortunately, the wave only grew. It grew so large that not even the best surfers on the planet would dare attempt to ride its dark crest. I had no idea what was going on, and only focused on pushing through, tolerating it. Suddenly, I noticed it was bathroom time.

Cringing, I thought, "No! Not now! I can't *move*!"

But time would only heighten my discomfort, and I was well aware of it. So, with Mom on one side and Nicholas on the other, I stood up, the world going fuzzy before clearing once again. I took my first step; ugh, this was going to take awhile. One by one, each foot made touchdown, and I took life millisecond by millisecond. A few times I had to stop and build up my strength for a minute or so before resuming the snaillike crawl. The two pegs that held me up, my legs, felt like they had never walked a day in their lives.

I concentrated unbelievably hard, my eyes focused on the bathroom door. At last, I made it. It had taken about five minutes, and when I arrived and plopped onto the toilet, my salvation, the relief that I felt was instantly incinerated by my exhaustion. Mom thanked Nicholas, and he went back to the living room and his computer.

After I had "taken care of business," as UPS puts it, my hand met my mom's, and together, we hoisted me up . . . it would have helped to have a pulley. Then, as I made a solo venture to the sink to wash up, tingling overcame me, my vision speckled, and my head spun. I stopped, and Mom looked at me.

"Are you okay?" she asked, her face displaying a hybrid mix of fright and concern.

Trying to pinpoint my problem, I could only blurt, "I feel dizzy . . . ," as I instantly blacked out.

I remember, quite clearly, a feeling like someone was pulling my brain up, up, up and out of my head. Dots in my vision divided and multiplied like cells, until I could see nothing. Mom said I was unconscious for about ten seconds, but oddly, I recall having a dream. It was about dancing . . . that's all I remember. I think I was at Kinderdance, where I used to take lessons when I started out at age three.

Next, the speckles faded out, until I could see the familiar bathroom tub in a foggy, blurry blob. Arms wrapped tightly around me, and I sat on a lap that trembled, as if in shock. Mom had caught me and, now, I sat on her lap as she sat atop the lid to the toilet. I recall mumbling, unable to speak comprehensible language. Wondering what had happened, I heard my shallow breathing, the thump, thump of my heart.

Mom still shook, and she now called out, "Nicholas! Nicholas!" as I remained slumped over in her lap.

There was no response, and she tried again. With me on top of her, the only way for her to go get help was for *both* of us to walk to the door and open it. What we didn't know, at the time, was that Nicholas was listening to music on his computer. He couldn't hear Mom's desperate cries. We were going to have to do it ourselves.

Then, Mom spoke to me. She told me I could take as much time as I needed, but that we just had to get to the door to open it, to call for help. I replied with a sort of mumble. So, for the next fifteen minutes, we sat on the toilet, Mom shaking, me barely conscious. I would have gotten up much sooner, but I physically could not. I truly thought I would die if I moved a single finger at that horrible moment in time. But, at last, Mom said we had to go, and I gathered one last umph of strength. Taking a deep breath, I slowly stood up. Mom grasped my arm, like we were magnets. I braced. It took so much power to have my legs hold me up, and I felt I could not lift my foot to take a single step.

But I began small, gaining about an inch every minute or so. The door, which stood less than ten feet away, mocked us. Mom's eyes went from me to the door, me to the door, and I stared off into some other dimension, attempting to summon strength from unknown forces. It was one of the most unbelievable feats I have ever accomplished.

I honestly thought, as I took each grueling step, "I don't know if I can do this."

But finally, as if in a game of Twister, Mom reached out for the doorknob, keeping a firm clasp on me as well. We had made it. Mom and I had done the impossible. We had walked to the bathroom door. Within moments, Nicholas appeared, his expression filled with shock and surprise. Mom still shook, and I felt bad for her.

The next thing I knew, I was in my brother's arms, being carried down the hall. I felt like a newborn, helpless, resting my head on his warm shoulder. Once again under the covers of my bed, I could have cried, but I was too tired. I was back . . . right back where I started.

Although much stronger than the previous day, I was still extremely weak the next morning. This was partly, I believe, because I was quite shaken up by the whole ordeal. One doesn't just leap back from traumatic events like that; it takes time to recover physically, and most of all, psychologically. I was overly cautious . . . prolonging each moment to be sure no sudden actions should trigger another fainting spell. A new appreciation glowed in my heart, as embers in a fire. Thankfulness was in my blood, sweat, tears, and, well . . . I won't go that far.

I was just finishing up my morning crossword puzzle as the telephone rang.

Mom answered it, greeting, "Good morning," in the same distinct way I have heard all of my life.

She later reenacted the call.

"A little birdie told me to call you," the voice of Dr. Dan announced.

Uh-oh. It was Dr. Dan.

"Why did the little birdie tell me to call you?" he asked.

Listening from the other room, I could tell that it was mostly a one-sided conversation. Occasionally, Mom broke in, blurting a few words in a defensive tone.

"If it concerns you, then it concerns me," Dr. Dan asserted.

Mom's voice rang with confusion and regret.

"Consider yourself admonished," was one of the last things she heard before setting the phone back on the receiver.

I giggled, Dr. Dan had "admonished" her. Someone at the office must have seen the post on my CarePage about me passing out, and he called to tell Mom that she should have called him. It strangely made me love him even more. The extent to which he cared went way beyond what Mom and I had ever expected.

We then knew that we could call for *anything*, and I joked, "Hey, Dr. Dan, just wanted to let you know I have to go to the bathroom!"

We both agreed that we'd better call him if we needed to in the future, or we'd get in trouble again.

❦

With a grunt, I executed a fluid pull-up on the chin-up bar in my parents' room. Then, like it was nothing, I cranked out two more. Actually, that's because it was nothing. Watching Nicholas do his nightly pull-ups, I had been counting them out for him like I usually did. A smile would crack on his red face as I played with him.

"One, two, three, two, three, four, two," I would announce, while tucked tightly into my mom's bed.

Shaking his head, he would just go along with it. This particular evening, when he completed a total of fifty or so, I could not help but play around with him.

"Mushy can do more than that!" I teased before breaking into an odd-sounding chuckle.

Maybe it was weird, because I knew in my heart that I definitely could not do a single pull-up. Gosh, I probably couldn't even walk to the chin-up bar.

Then Nicholas, who looked at me with empathy, asked, "Mushy, do you want to do a pull-up?"

Before I even had time to think of how I was feeling, I was climbing out of bed. I sure wasn't gonna miss out on a little fun. Having done some, well, not-so-fun stuff for the past few months, I thought that I deserved a little. This was my chance. Shuffling under the doorway, Nicholas stood behind me. I reached up, feeling sharp pains from the Neupogen shots but, at that moment, I didn't give a darn. Grasping the bar, I suddenly lifted into the air and hovered just off the ground.

So, there I was, in the strong hold of my brother's arms, moving up and down as if I was the one doing them. Thinking back to that evening, the one just after the dreadful events of post-chemo, I see symbolism in the image of Nicholas and me. I pulled up with all of my might but, without my brother, I would have never reached the top. This is akin to my journey. I pulled, I climbed, and I fought . . . but I wouldn't have gotten really anywhere without all of the people who love me underneath, pushing my butt. Thanks guys, and sorry if I farted.

I grabbed a nice, fluffy pillow. Whack! The sound it made as it smacked my brother was worse than it actually was. After completing my pull-ups, I had gone back to bed, only to start a pillow fight with Dean. Of course, it was a one-way pillow fight, with Dean not about to hit his cancer-ridden sister with a pillow.

As I gave him "love smacks," he whirled around and told me, "Wow, Mushy, you have energy!"

Hmm . . . I hadn't really thought about it, but yeah . . . I guess it was so. I felt terrible physically, so it must have been joy. I had not had that much fun in a *long* time, and my gratitude filtered into pure *happiness*. Life is meant to be fun, and when something is trying to prevent us from having some, it gets really tough. But nothing can ever prevent us from making a good time. It's all in our attitude.

One can be sentenced to life in prison and decide, "You know, I'm gonna make this fun."

It's drastic, but it can happen. I truly believe that people in the world don't have as much fun as they should. This is because most of them think that fun comes to them and that others are responsible for their fun and enjoyment. Bzzzzzz! Wrong! Fun, happiness, love . . . you name it, it's created by us, and *only* us. Many people complain and complain about something being "no fun" or "boring." Heck! Do something about it. Sometimes I look at our society and think that people *enjoy* complaining about stuff. Rather than take action to resolve their personal crisis, they rant and rave, getting absolutely *nowhere* productive.

The way I see it, we're here, right? We only have so much time here on Earth, and I don't think you, me, or the next guy yearns to watch you sulk through your whole life story in Heaven's Movie Theater. I know I would walk out. Each moment should be fun and not judged by what we are *doing*.

For example, a root canal, a colonoscopy, or chemo are not fun all by themselves, but *one* who is having a good time and glows with happiness can diminish all of the myths about stuff *having* to be "not fun." I then realized, as I gave my bro one last whack, that I had the power to spontaneously, and randomly, produce fun and joy from scratch. Who says a girl with cancer can't have fun?

⌒

Looking into Larry's loving, soft, golden-brown eyes, I celebrated a victory for Team Melinda and Jaynie. The Let-Larry-on-the-Bed Campaign was a success, that is, after much pestering of and pleading to the other party, aka, Dad. We settled on a nice compromise, with a protective sheet having to be placed on top of the bed upon Larry's arrival.

Things were always great when he was cuddled next to me, his excess skin making him all the more "mooshable." The look on his face told me that he understood everything, and a new, rare gentleness came over him.

Slowly, he would give his paw to me, almost as if to ask, "Are you okay?"

With his ears nearly back to his bottom, he stared at me with the sweetest, most compassionate expression on Earth.

Occasionally, he would want to get playful with me, but that being too rough, I would ask him calmly, "Do you want to get down, Larry? If you want to be rough, you have to get down."

Like a scolded child, he instantly behaved, with a look of rue present on his adorable face. Some of the best moments I remember with Larry were when I would cry.

On rough mornings, when the prednisone didn't go down too well, or I was just plain sick of being sick, Mom would ask me, "Do you *need* him?"

Of course, the answer was always, "Yes."

So, bounding in, he would leap onto the bed, not only his tail but also his entire rump whipping in a circular pattern. After he settled down, his warm, soft body against mine made everything better. I stroked him softly. The way he breathed against me was relaxing. I pet him, I hugged him, and I kissed him, and he just soaked it all up like a mop—a big, yellow, furry mop. Larry has always been very sensitive, so when he saw me cry, he knew something was terribly wrong. He would stare at me, his eyes worried and confused. I believe he was somewhat frustrated that he couldn't really do anything. But he *was* doing something. He was just being there. His calm aura brought serenity *and* sanity back to my rotting soul.

Sometimes, it's nice to be with someone, or something, who just *listens*, and in Larry's case, he had no choice but to sit there and listen to me. But I think he genuinely wanted to listen . . . because he cared about his little Melinda. Dogs are one of the most sacrificial animals . . . you give them a bed and food . . . and in return, you get their eternal, unconditional love.

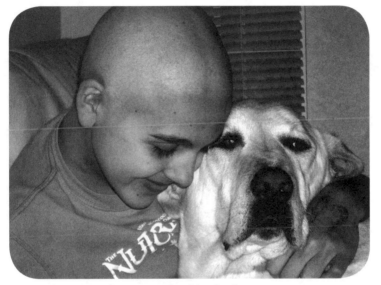

A moment of nothing but love . . .

"Lots of people talk to animals . . . Not very many listen, though . . . That's the problem." —Benjamin Hoff

ELEVEN

"I'M BALD!" I exclaimed, just moments after I recovered from a sleep-induced unconsciousness.

Being in rare form, I rubbed the little prickles that still clung on my head. My mom, who had awakened at the exact same moment as I, started her morning off with a good laugh. And as the day progressed, it proved to be a better day, a more exciting day, and an all-around easier day.

Amalia came to draw labs, while I once again braced—helplessly pinned down on the bed by the needle hovering above me. Knowing that I had already done it once helped, because I knew what to expect and what discomfort I would experience. Amalia checked my pulse and listened to my lungs. Everything was good, except for her slight concern about my blood pressure being very low. After promising to drink plenty of fluids to maintain my body's balance, I watched as Amalia's car door slammed and she drove off down the street.

Nurse Pam called. It was later that afternoon, and she already brought good news from my blood test results. My counts had come up enough so that they were almost back to normal. We could discontinue the shots.

"Yay, one less poke," I thought.

Laughing, I felt relief. It was a small victory, but it added a drop into the millions of drops in the ocean of healing. Without that one drop, it would be smaller. But there was an even greater victory in the making. I had the green light. I could go to dance. Realizing that I was far away from physically being able to dance, Mom and I agreed on a compromise. I would watch. My spirit, an arid riverbed, was flooded and rejuvenated by my excitement and joy. Nearly crying, I slipped on my beanie and prepared to go. Even though I wouldn't *dance*, I didn't care. I was going . . . and that's all that mattered.

⌒

"Melinda!" the dancers screamed as I entered the hall just outside the studio.

Happy to see them as well, I was overtaken with a wave of hugs—one after another.

One girl asked, "How was your Christmas?"

Not exactly knowing how to reply, but appreciating her thoughtfulness, I simply replied, "Busy," while chuckling under my breath.

I sat down amid the dozens of dance bags and stinky *pointe* shoes . . . it felt great. Looking around, I saw that everything was the same. Everyone was there. Imagining what things would be like, when I would—finally—return to class, I pictured it all very different. I envied the other girls because of their health and their ability to dance. But it was a unique kind of envy that gave off feelings of joy for them, not bad feelings of any sort.

The class before us ended, and a herd of sweaty little girls ran into their moms' waiting arms. My fellow dancers loaded up their bags and made their way in against the flow of the few lagging smaller girls. I had my cell phone and a water bottle. I stood back, afraid to get caught up in a crowd of people and, therefore, *germs*.

As I ventured back into my natural habitat, the studio, surprise shone on my teacher's face. Hugging Ms. Cynthia, I could feel the genuine care she possessed for me. After informing her that I would be just watching, my bottom hit the dance floor, and I leaned against the massive mirrors up front. I could see everything: the long, wall-length *barres*, the doors, the music box. I was in heaven. And when that beautiful, soft song began to hum for *pliés*, it did something for my soul. I was practically doing the movements, only it was just my spirit doing them, feeling the music with a new energy and passion.

The short hour I was there sped by faster than a Concorde Jet. Although I was thrilled to watch and to be well enough to go, there was a sadness that ticked in me—it was a weird combo. I longed for the feeling of dancing, the feeling of freedom, the feeling of the studio air filling my lungs, and the feeling of my heart beating as one with the music. I decided I would work hard. I would do it . . . I would dance again. The fear of hard work did not exist within me. Becoming accustomed to pain, I now didn't care one bit how badly anything hurt.

I always told myself, "It's just pain . . . it's just pain."

In a way, it was great that I could disconnect from my bodily discomfort, but at the same time, I was almost becoming *too* used to it. I almost didn't care. Convinced that I was made to suffer, I began to dislike my body and borderline hate it. It didn't matter what *it* went through, but only what *I* went through. And as I watched my friends dance across the floor before my eyes, I planned a major comeback. My initial thought was doubt-filled, but in my heart, I was determined to become an even greater dancer than before.

Bent over like a ninety-year-old, I hobbled with Mom's help toward my bed. Despite my Hunchback-like appearance, I was full of spunk, on a high from going to watch dance class.

"They did this *really cool* combination!" I told Mom. "Do you want to see it?"

Her face read both "yes," and "no," but after I reassured her that I would be cautious, she stepped aside. Hitting a beautiful and perfect fifth position, I smiled. It felt *so good*. Then, I began. Like an old car warming up, I slowly skated along the floor with pitiful jumps and footwork. Landing in fourth position, I pushed off with all of my might and executed the absolute slowest, most sluggish *pirouette* of my life.

Mom beamed, a special light glowing in her eyes that seemed to come straight from her heart. Helping me into bed, she saw my peaceful smile. I was exhausted, but the dance endorphins in my brain popped and crackled like fireworks. My heart beat fast . . . it felt right. I had danced equivalent to how I danced at age three, and every single step was pretty much a disgrace to the dance world. But the joy that came from those hideous few steps was a kind of happiness that came only from dancing. My body *needs* to move, and I went to sleep that night with the sensation that I had finally gotten something out of my system.

The tribal-like music blared, and my body strained to do the movements. I was actually doing it . . . what I thought was entirely impossible . . . I was dancing. On the brink of crying out of joy, I was distracted by the intense concentration it took to make my body do what I begged it to accomplish. Tuesday was modern class, and my bald head had an almost internal glow under the dim lights.

I felt horrible. My vision was fuzzy, my legs were weaker than twigs, and my back moaned with the intense pain from the Neupogen shots. But somehow I kept going. As long as the music was playing, it carried me, supported me. I didn't think. The music and my spirit guided my body through every single step.

The most amazing feeling on Earth is when I am just dancing, not thinking, stressing, or trying too hard to control the movements. It was happiness, and my love for dance, that moved me and kept me going. Experiencing a new, powerful connection with the melodic beat of the song, I felt like I was in a dream . . . it was too good to be true. Having virtually no coordination, God moved me, like His little puppet. Somehow managing to make my fragile body appear graceful, I danced in honor of life and Him.

Slowly, I hobbled over to the waiting piano bench. Once settled, my shaking hands began to skim over the ivory keys, and a beautiful tune echoed throughout the house. I could see the reflection of my head in the slick, black shine of our Steinway Grand. To be honest, I didn't even remember how to play the song, but my fingers just knew where to go, what to do. It had been months since I played. The song was "Can't Help Falling in Love with You," by Elvis Presley. It was my mom's favorite of the songs that I played—and I believe it still is.

Exactly like I had done previously that evening in dance class, my heart and the music fused, like plugging an extension cord into a power strip. Love and hope poured out of every note, and the piano never sounded so exquisite. Out of the corner of my eye, I saw Mom. She stood at the kitchen sink, peeling an apple. With a soft smile, I watched as her tears flowed down, landing in the small pile of peelings.

Dance. The following day was again filled with dance. I was thrilled to announce to Mom, as we drove home from class, that I had done all but one combination at *barre*. Then I bragged about how I drank a whole bottle of water. Dr. Dan, Amalia, and Mom had all been on me about ingesting more fluids since the fainting episode, and I felt like they would be proud of me.

After *barre*, I watched the rest of class.

With my "dome" gleaming under the bright studio lights, one girl commented, "Wow, you never really realize how tan you are until you don't have any hair!"

It was true. A white "cap" displayed itself atop my head, where my hair had once lived. Where my part had been, a tan stripe paved its way from front to back. We all ended up laughing. It felt good to make fun of myself. We're not a whole person if we don't laugh at ourselves once in awhile. We giggled with the rest of the class about my "white swim cap," joking that I should get a spray tan on my head.

⌒

"You know, I really feel like some tasty oral contrast," I groaned, sarcastically, at the breakfast table.

A chest X-ray, as well as a PET/CT scan, was scheduled for later on that day. What seemed like only minutes after I said this, it became a reality. Sitting in the radiology waiting room, I pounded down bottle number two of the acrid, chalky substance. Then I routinely went test hopping from X-ray to scanner. I was becoming good at it. Ha ... funny thing to be good at.

Results. They're what everyone in this world waits for, hopes for, and works for. And boy, did we get them. The PET scan was entirely normal, with no hot spots of cancerous activity. Also, the CT scan brought on some God-praising news. My mass had decreased 50 percent! That's right ... one half of it. Whoosh! Gone. This was amazing. After two rounds, half of it had disappeared. I added it up in my head. If two rounds equaled 50 percent, then four rounds equals 100 percent. If, that is, it kept decreasing at the same rate. Hoping, thanking, praising, and praying all at once, I fell into a strange kind of sleep. And just before I drifted off, I giggled—my head was cold. I slipped on my warmest beanie; God closed my eyes and let me rest.

Mom entered the room with pods of tears in her eyes. I could see that they were not sad tears, because the feeling was different—their presence was different. I was right. The exciting news Mom brought poked at my soul. A dear friend, Debi Miller, was going to run in a 10K race to raise money for a children's hospital in Arizona.

Not only that, but she told Mom, "I'm going to wear a photo of Melinda proudly pinned to my shirt."

The tears just came. They were unexpected tears, but good, cleansing tears. I then realized that my illness created these kinds of opportunities and moments in time. Flowing down my cheeks, my tears represented the happy side of cancer.

My feet rapidly shuffled around my room, and a dust cloth whipped here and there. I called my brothers and then watched as they muscled my heavy dresser to the opposite wall. I wanted it changed. *All changed.* Everything would be cleaned and changed, if it was the last thing I did. I was sick of my old room, the one I had, for so long, cried in, prayed in, and pleaded in. I couldn't bring myself to lie in the same spot, staring at the same things as I did before. Things were different now. I was getting better, and I wanted change . . . *now.*

After tidying up my desk, I collapsed onto my bed. I opened my eyes to observe my work. Looking around, I barely recognized my room. It had a new and strange feeling. Crud.

Run ragged from the previous day, I was too exhausted and light-headed to go to dance class. "Rough" kept proving to be my motto of the day. In fact, as soon as I rose from bed, I knew instantly the day was going to beat me up, take my lunch money, and throw me in a dumpster. Grabbing my robe, I headed for the bathroom. I went to sit down . . . slosh . . . the end of my long robe dragged into the toilet. Half whining, half laughing, I located Mom and told her what had happened.

"I'm having a Robe in the Toilet Day!"

Ah, it was going to be a long day. Now, whenever Mom or I, or both of us, have a day that bites us in the rump, we declare it a *Robe in the Toilet Day*.

Huddled on the couch, I created a giant, hexagonal-shaped, 3-D origami structure. Origami had become another one of my mind-numbing activities.

I was getting sick of making tiny boxes and pyramids out of little strips of paper, so I decided, "Hey! Why not get giant pieces of paper and make the same thing?"

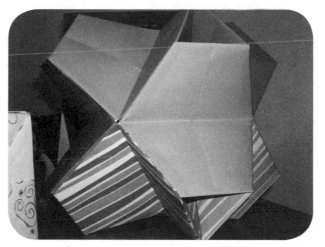

One of my giant origami masterpieces!

With an array of colored papers burying me alive, I repeated the same motion over and over and over. Fold, crease, fold, crease. My fingers turned red and became irritated, but I just kept going. Fold, crease, fold, crease. My hands were still working, while my conscience was in a far-off place. The doorbell rang, snapping me out of Origami Land. I got excited over the silliest things when I was sick . . . stuff that other people, normal people, would think was stupid. The harmonic tone of our doorbell was one of those things. I saw the faint blur of a man in brown shorts and work boots. Oh, boy . . . UPS.

The odd-shaped package fell into my hands as I stared at it with curiosity. Ripping it open with the utmost carelessness, I extracted an envelope with my first and last name formally, and beautifully, written on the front. I tore it open and began to decipher the neat and perfect cursive message. I read words, but I didn't exactly process them. I skipped to the bottom.

Amazed, I finally realized it was signed "*Patricia Barker.*"

My hands began to shake, and my eyes became two glaciers, melting and forming rivers upon my cheeks.

Patricia Barker . . . oh my gosh. I had watched her farewell performance at the Pacific Northwest Ballet in Seattle the previous June, in celebration of my thirteenth birthday. She inspired me. Her fluidity, musicality, and strength left me in awe. I was stunned by her grace . . . inside and out. Gasping for breath, I looked to Mom. I remained speechless. There were no words, truly, no words.

Soaking up the beautiful moment, I realized that cancer had created it. Well, not cancer *itself*, but me having it. It was these times that I saw the other side of cancer. I knew I would not be standing there—my body numb, my eyes gushing, and that letter in my hands—if not for it. Cancer is battle after battle, struggle after struggle. And then, something beautiful happens that keeps you going.

Venturing back into the package, my hand met something hard. The object was not in view, but I knew, from the feel and shape, exactly what it was. The only thing was . . . I didn't believe it. My mind wouldn't let me. Delicately pulling the precious gift from its royal sheath, a flash flood occurred in my eyeballs. It was *pointe* shoes . . . *her pointe* shoes.

"*To Melinda*" was visible on the tip of one shoe.

A gold ribbon tied the two slippers together, creating an almost angelic presentation. I held them as if they were gold . . . they meant even more than gold to me. With my tears continuing to flow, I stared at what sat in my unworthy hands. I looked at them from all angles. They were incredible. Examining the bottom, I read the small writing on each shoe.

"*Barker, Swan Lake, Act II*"

Oh my gosh. My heart pounded. I could not believe what was happening to me. After suffering so much, I almost felt it was too good to be true, like I didn't deserve it or anything. My mouth hung open, my breathing was awkward, and my face was hot and red from crying. I lost it—completely lost it. Burying my head in my arms, I cried so hard that it hurt. Never had anything touched me in such a way. To hear encouragement to keep fighting from someone who I admired was breathtakingly unimaginable.

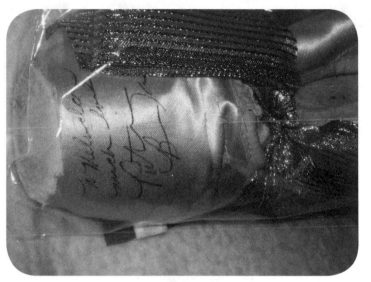

THE shoes.

Her letter was filled with wisdom, hope, and an understanding of what it is like to have a hindrance affect the dance in your life. She also told me that when I beat cancer, I would dance again with a new love and passion. Her certainty made me believe her and gave me a ray of light in the view of my future.

She concluded by saying, "I will look for you on the big stage of life."

Ms. Barker, your words are eloquent, and they've had a huge impact on my life. What you did for me will forever remain in my heart.

That night, I drifted off into a tranquil sleep, with *the* shoes wrapped tightly in my arms . . . perfectly preserved in a large Ziploc bag. I hugged them all night long.

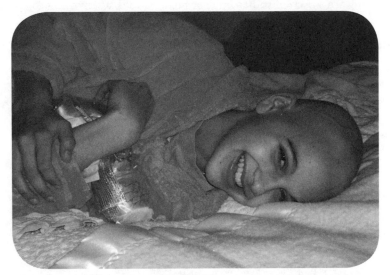

Good night . . .

"When you win your battle with cancer you will dance again and you will bring a new spirit and passion with you because of what you have gone through and overcome." —Patricia Barker

TWELVE

"I WANT TO BE done *right now*," I complained.

I was going through a phase. It was a phase of realization that I could not just wave a magic wand and be done. I had a long way to go, and thinking about it frustrated me to the core. Patience. Patience was the name of the game, and unfortunately, I was not very good at that game. We need so much of it in this life, and the multitudes of us do not practice patience as often as we should. We are an anxious, impatient species . . . *far* from perfect. I'm human. I got crabby, tired, overwhelmed, and impatient with my plight. However, my humor wiggled through even the smallest of spaces. Random expressions of my near insanity became a regular thing.

One day, as I noticed tiny, prickly hairs regrowing on my head, I asked Mom, out of the blue, "I'm getting a 5 o'clock shadow on my head! Can you please get me some Aveeno Lotion for my dome?"

Yep, it seemed that if I wasn't crying, I was laughing. One particular comical incident I remember quite well. Mom and I were on our way home in the car, and we slid to a stop at the giant blue mailbox in front of our post office. Rolling down my window, I stretched out like a giraffe reaching for a leafy dinner. Plop! The envelopes fell in and disappeared. Just then, a lady who works at the post office, who we have known for years, came strolling out with a large container to collect the pile of mail.

My first thought was, "Look! It's Debbie!"

But then I recalled that my appearance was *slightly* different from when I'd seen her last.

"Oh crap! I'm bald!" I cried, fumbling for my beanie.

She neared the box—everything seemed like it was *National Geographic* slow. Not wanting to explain my whole story in my exhausted state, I scrambled, found my hat, and jammed it in an awkward way atop my head. Mom found an opening in the traffic, and we zoomed away. I felt like Mrs. James Bond.

Scream laughter erupted from Mom and me. That was a close one. There were times when we cried together, there were times when we laughed together, and there were times when we laughed *and* cried together. This was one of those moments.

⌒

I awoke February ninth to a bright, sunny, warm, glorious day that God had made. But God made something even more beautiful on that day in the past . . . my mom. It was her birthday, and although none of us was expecting me to be in my then present state, it was a fun, memorable day.

Enjoying the warm sun in our pool area, I grabbed the bottle of sunscreen. I held it high above my head and squeezed a good amount onto my delicate dome. Sunburn would not be good. Reaching to rub it in, I discovered a mountain of white goop atop my dome. Nicholas was nearby, and together we eventually worked it all in—after some vigorous rubbing. Ha, ha, it tickled. Then I was ready to be outside in God's incredible day. It was something I had not done in a very long while, and I didn't know how much I had missed it until I rocked in the hammock under our maple tree, gazing up at the bright blue sky.

That night, we went to dinner. It was a nice restaurant, and I slipped on what I considered "nice, but comfy." Christmas was the last time I had gone near my nicer clothes, because my pajama drawer had been frequented for the past couple of months. This was also the first time I was out, exposed in public—among normal people.

Concerned about the reactions that would surface, I wondered—not about how others' reactions would affect *me*, but how my startling appearance would affect *others*. I didn't care about how *I* looked; I was mainly apprehensive that no one in the entire restaurant would be able to choke down their linguini and clams with me around. After wearing my pink fuzzy beanie for quite some time, I became hot—hot enough to buy a salmon fillet and grill it on my head.

Turning to Mom, I asked, "Should I take it off?"

Tugging at the top of my hat, I so badly wished to rip it off, free my head, and let the cool air refresh me. But I looked around the room with uncertainty . . . what would people think? Would everyone stare, or make a conscious effort to ignore me? I wanted neither. Becoming exhausted, I realized that I was over-thinking things *way* too much. I didn't care anymore; I popped it off. Pausing, I almost expected an uproar of shock, complete with gasps and screams. But everything remained exactly the same, with nothing but the soft hum of con-versations, the clanging of forks on plates, and the occasional sizzle echoing out from the kitchen. I glanced across the table at my mom. I felt bad for, well, not ruining her birthday, but making it . . . well . . . different.

On February 11, 2008, two days after Mom's birthday, Round 3 of Melinda vs. Hodgkin lymphoma took place. Millions across the world ordered it in HD and were glued to their flat screens. Nah . . . just kidding. I entered to find a spacious, private room awaiting my arrival. The bed was neatly made, the dry erase board displayed my name, and my pink bucket was elaborately decorated with layers of glittery stickers. I thought it was sweet of them to do that for me, although I wished the whole bucket thing would be entirely unnecessary in the first place.

I, too, came bearing surprises. Gift bags weighed down my arms. I had asked what people's favorite colors were during my previous round, and I had been busily knitting away, creating personalized scarves for each one. A heavenly presence filled my spirit as I watched smile after smile appear on the faces of the recipients. Only giving could create that instantaneous spurt of joy in my soul . . . and I treasured it.

They checked me in, and weird, uncomfortable questions began . . . same old, same old. From my bed, I felt like I had a panoramic view of all of Santa Bar-bara. The mountains looked spectacular and prominent in the evening sun, and Santa Barbara Mission glowed with a calm peacefulness. I could stare out at it all day . . . practically did.

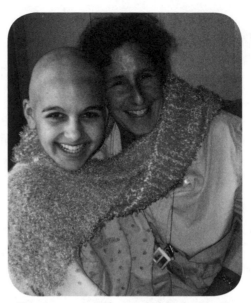

Keeping warm in the scarf I knit for Jaynie.

Earlier, I had joked with Mom about what I was giving her for her birth-day. "I'm going to pamper you with a two-night stay at the luxurious Cottage Hospital."

Giggling, I realized that all I had promised her was there. I don't know how, but it was. As my first bag of chemo was strung up, I gazed out at the outside world, wondering what other people were doing. They were driving home from work, putting the kids to bed, maybe swinging through Mickey D's for dinner, getting chemo. Oh no . . . wait. That was just me.

It was a Tuesday night, and you know what that meant. It meant *American Idol* with Mom. Their famous "Da da da da da da da, DA DA!" rang as Mom snug-gled behind me on my bed. She wrapped her arms around me, and that was it. I couldn't have dreamed of being in a better place at that moment. Disregarding the bag of chemo dripping into me, everything was perfect, calm, and heavenly.

There's something about when someone hugs you. They feel unnaturally warm, and this warmth melts away any pain that you have. Their love burns a fire that creates this toastiness, and their embrace is the closest thing they can do to jumping in your body and doing it for you. Serenity. It was pure serenity as Mom held me in her arms. I hoped that she would never let go and that the moment would last forever.

But of course, "All good things must come to an end."

About fifteen or twenty minutes into *American Idol*, I began to feel extremely dizzy, tired, and nauseated. As they cut to a commercial break, I decided to close my eyes and rest for a minute or so. Bad idea. I was out like a light the very second my eyelids closed. Sleeping into fathoms of depth I hadn't reached in sleep for a long time, I finally awoke, my bladder sending out SOS signals. It was dark . . . really dark . . . like one o'clock in the morning dark.

With my best chemo chuckle, I concluded, "Hmm . . . must've dozed off."

❦

My blood pressure was low, alarmingly so. Mom now admits to me that, as I slept, her eyes remained permanently glued to my monitor, with a quick, periodic glance at me now and again. Even Dr. Dan was concerned. And so, I watched as a large, upside down bottle of Albumin was hung alongside my fresh, new bag of fluids. Extremely what I like to call "chemoed-out," I wasn't exactly sure what it was, but only that it was supposed to help me. Looking up at it, I found it resembled . . . champagne. Its slightly bubbly appearance, along with my unintentional drunken stupor, was quite a sight.

Jaynie wheeled me, and Mom pushed my IV pole . . . aka Ricco. The patio was our destination, and I smiled at nurses and other folks as we rolled past. Soaring straight up, the elevator delivered and spit us out at the top floor. After my wheelchair and equipment were jammed through the small doorway, I was struck with the fresh, pure outside air. It was as clear as glass and as crisp as a potato chip.

I instantly felt more awake, healthy, and, well . . . more *alive*. Something about the outdoors really gets me. When I experience a beautiful moment in nature, it brings me closer to the Earth. It makes me feel more natural, which is exactly what I needed to cope with the horrible, toxic chemicals that then polluted me. Being outside brings me closer to God. He made this amazing planet for us to enjoy, and many of us don't stop and truly soak up its peace, its love, and its tranquility. But there's something about lying in the bland hospital, with nothing but the smell of non-latex gloves and bad cafeteria food, that can change a person.

The gentle breeze and warm sun captivated my senses. As I sat in my wheelchair, indirectly drinking my champagne, I gazed with wonder on what God made . . . and rediscovered the world all over again.

☞

Dogs, dogs, and more dogs . . . my third round was Dog Round. Jaynie knew just how much I loved visits from the many therapy dogs, so with one quick phone call, I nearly had dogs lining up at my door. Echo, Scruffy, Carmel, Dottie, and Ralph all came to cheer me, with lolling tongues and wagging tails.

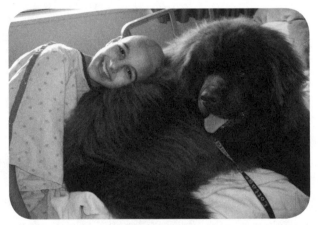

Me and Echo the therapy bear . . . oh, I mean dog.

And then . . . there was Rowan. Rowan is Jaynie's registered therapy dog, a 122-pound Leonberger, with just as much love as fur. Of course, Rowan not only had to be *on* the bed with me, but *on top* of me. Her giant tongue painted my face with a layer of slobber. Ah . . . I loved it.

She wore a bandana that read, "I didn't ask to be a princess, but if the tiara fits . . ."

Her giant paws were as big as my feet, and in terms of pounds, Melinda + Melinda = Rowan. Her huge, gentle, compassionate eyes stared not only into my eyes but into my heart. Gathering virtually all of the nurses on Peds, and visiting faithful friend Casey, we posed for a classic Kodak moment. A crowd of smiling faces surrounded my bed, and lost in a sea of Rowan fur was little Melinda.

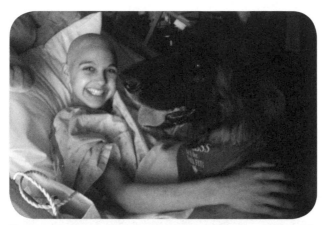

Rowan gives me slobber, fur, and love during chemo Round 3.

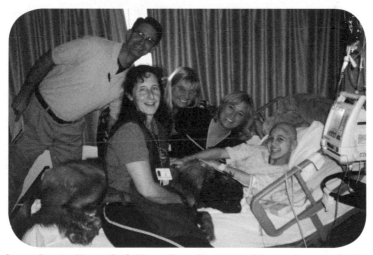

Casey, Jaynie, Nurse Gail, Nurse Pam, Rowan, and I pose for a quick shot.

Jaynie and I had a lot of fun my third round. One morning, we watched the *Eukanuba Dog Show* on TV for hours, laughing and sharing our love for the adorable critters. Jaynies's pager would sound, but with the push of one button, we were once again entranced by the show. Third round fun also came in the form of art. Supplies and blank paper were transformed into anything my chemo-controlled mind could think of.

I vividly remember asking Jaynie, shortly after my arrival, "What do you think I should draw?"

An open marker was gripped in my hand, ready to create the next masterpiece.

"Something symbolic," she suggested, giving me a high-eyebrow look.

With that, I took off. Not long passed, and I set down my last marker. It was beautifully disturbing: lovely, yet mysterious; peaceful, yet creepy. It was the bottom of the ocean. Half of the paper was dark and eerie, with a lifeless blob slowly sinking to the bottom. It was my mass. It was cancer. The upper portion was composed of a bright, golden sunset, a leaping dolphin, colorful flowers, and bright pink, *pointe* shoe clouds. I believed it was one of my finest works while in the hospital, that is, my best *drawing*.

My art was also displayed through other mediums, such as clay. I sculpted a little doctor bear sitting on a heart platform for Dr. Dan. His name spanned the back of the bear's doctor coat, and I don't mean to brag, but it was pretty adorable, and I was the proud Picasso.

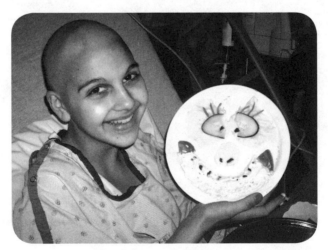

Hospitals can get boring . . .

Clay and paper were not my only forms of expression; there was food as well. Yes, food. Okay, okay, I know every mom teaches her children not to play with food, but really, come on! It's fun! You've gotta do something with those leftovers, you know? So I would create a face on my plate. Mashed potatoes became eyes, tomatoes lips, and cereal teeth. It was stress relief and amusement wrapped up in one hysterical package. It was exactly what one would expect coming from me. It was so Melinda.

◔

The fun and joy were there and gone. They popped in and out like a bunny out of a magician's hat. Rough moments, minutes, hours, and days still occurred, and I took them on with a slow and steady strength. I can still recall the episode of *SpongeBob* that played as Dr. Dan entered my private suite to check up on me. Suddenly, belly laughter gurgled out of me. Patrick the Starfish was in his underwear. Startled, Dr. Dan stared at me, with a face of 50 percent surprise and 50 percent confusion.

"I'm sorry. I'm sorry," I gasped through my laughter attack.

"It's just . . . Patrick's in his underwear!" I blurted, pointing up at the screen.

After turning to view the TV, Dr. Dan looked back to me, smiling and shaking his head as if he couldn't quite believe me. I think he hasn't really had any patients like me. With Patrick then dressed, and my laughter ebbing, the mood suddenly shifted in the room. It was time to get down to business.

After a brief examination, Dr. Dan drew up a seat beside my bed. I could tell by his expression that he was serious, and it startled me a little. I didn't like it when Dr. Dan was serious. He calmly told me, in his Pediatric Voice, that although the Albumin helped my blood pressure, there was a strong chance that, because of my very low blood counts, I would need a transfusion.

The word flew out and cut me. I began to cry. I'm not sure why it got to me the way it did, but I believe that "transfusion" referring to me was a little much to handle. I wanted my own blood and nothing but mine.

"Why does that scare you?" I remember Dr. Dan asking.

Distressed, I replied honestly, "I don't know."

◔

During my stay, the hours crawled at an excruciating pace, but, as I looked for the last time at the view from my room, it seemed it had flown by. My various stuffed animal friends and I relaxed back in my wheelchair, waving to all of my friends at the nurse's station as we made our grand exit out the double doors. I was out. It felt like I had just used my Get out of Jail Free Card in a real-life game of Monopoly.

We entered into the hospital lobby, where a woman stopped us just before we reached the sliding doors. Mom had left to get the car and pull it around, so only Nurse Gail and I were there. A bright smile displayed itself prominently on the tall woman's face. I thought she was only being nice by grinning, but then she spoke.

"Do you know what day it is tomorrow?" she asked.

Flipping the calendar inside my head, I found February, and replied, "Valentine's Day?"

"Yes, you're right," she told me.

Her voice had a sweet tone, and was infused with an accent I couldn't identify. Then she reached out her hand. In it lay a small necklace with a large heart, dangling gracefully.

"I bought this for someone very special. I want to give my heart to you," she recited meaningfully.

Placing it in my hand, she twisted a small wheel on the back of it. The heart lit up, and so did mine. I felt numb. All was quiet.

Staring at the glowing necklace, words would not escape me until I found a quiet, soft, "Wow, thank you."

The necklace was just a *thing*, but this woman was a *real* person, with *real* love in her spirit. And just like that, she was gone, vanished down one of the identical hallways of the hospital. She was like an angel . . . there and gone. She spread her love, her joy, and God's grace, and whoosh! She was not there anymore. I clung tightly onto that necklace for a long while after. It wasn't until I finally let go that I noticed the small heart shape pressed into my palm.

"I expect to pass through this life but once. If, therefore, there be any kindness I can show, or any good thing I can do for any other fellow being, let me do it now, for I shall not pass this way again."
—William Penn

THIRTEEN

AFTER EACH ROUND, I would return home to a mountain of pills. I was literally drowning in them and, unfortunately, I didn't have the luxury of having them administered intravenously, like in the hospital. We invested in a pill cutter, and each morning, I would chop every prednisone tablet into four perfect wedges. I didn't know what would be worse, three big ones, or twelve tiny ones. I opted for tiny.

Also greeting me as I reached home was Bactrim. This giant Horse Pill was the granddaddy of them all.

I exclaimed, "It's as big as a TV remote and tastes like one too."

These I would crush. Dreading my Bactrim on weekend mornings and evenings, I would mentally prepare before dumping it all into a vanilla Ensure shake, swallowing, shivering, and gagging simultaneously. It always took a little while before full recovery took place and the bitter taste had completely diminished. The only thing which, sort of, comforted me was that it protected me from a life-threatening kind of pneumonia . . . which I was very susceptible to with my extremely weak immune system. I would get pretty irritable and upset over taking it, but all it took was Dr. Dan offering me the liquid form to put me back in my place.

Observing my Pill Courses at breakfast, I noticed a new item added to the menu . . . Florinef. Florinef was to help me maintain a steady fluid balance and, therefore, assist me in being less light-headed. It was small, oval, and yellow . . . an innocent-looking thing. But it was still a drug . . . *another* drug inside of me.

It's hard relying on unwanted substances to keep you, well, basically . . . alive. I wanted to stop *everything* right then, but I couldn't. My body was now used to it—needed it.

⤳

Cupid arrived on my doorstep . . . well, actually, my friend Ivana. A small bug stuffed animal, sitting on a box of heart candy, was clutched in her palms. Excited to see her, I also felt sort of bad for not being the easiest thing to look at. She wore a wide smile, and her sweetness touched me. Just to know that she thought of me lying there, struggling, made it that much easier. And, although I didn't want people constantly worrying about me, their thoughts and prayers created an invisible army around me.

More Valentine surprises came. A small, plush SpongeBob popped out of a package. His buck-toothed smile made me smile, and that smile only broadened as I saw a note, written in black Sharpie, on the back.

"Ahoy, Melinda. Tom Kenny."

It was him . . . SpongeBob—oh, actually, the *voice* of SpongeBob. My uncle knows Tom Kenny because he gets his mail at the same place. I was loved, loved by everyone. With the support I was receiving, there was nothing that could happen but healing, nowhere to go but up. Staring at the little yellow Sponge-Bob gripped in my hands, I felt it was yet another symbol of the outside encouragement and love I was receiving. It reminded me to appreciate friends and family who gave me a boost. They were my pulley—my springboard. They were my wings while I grew my own back.

⤳

I was either feeling better or just not caring anymore . . . I'm not sure which. Three days after reaching home, I was out of bed, busy baking breadsticks and cookies. Pulling energy from the reserves of my reserves, I motored around the kitchen before plopping down, once again, in my bed. Cooking and baking were therapeutic for me, and although I crashed, exhausted, afterward, some sort of happy, culinary sensation crackled inside of me. Also keeping me busy, and distracted from Cancerpalooza, were knitting and even writing stories for my schoolwork. Desperately searching for sources of mind-numbing activities, I became frustrated when I was too sick to be distracted, when I just had to *lie there* . . . ugh.

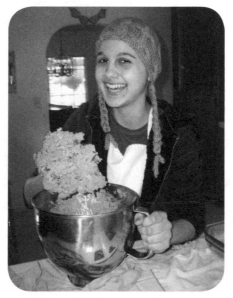

Cookies anyone?

Different events throughout my illness picked me up and pushed me down. Receiving news of other sick family and friends opened a special valve in my heart, and compassion gushed everywhere. Great-Aunt Marion, Great-Aunt Phyllis, Great-Uncle Abbott, and our dear friend Priscilla were all having their own health challenges. I was saddened but, at the same time, enjoyed the deep understanding that I then had for them. We were all peers—all on the same level. And although each one of our situations was different, I almost felt like I belonged to a special "club"—a "brotherhood" and a "sisterhood."

Danish pastries slid into the oven . . . *yum*. I was in a droopy and nauseous phase, in dire need of distraction. Even if that distraction came in the form of a piece of yarn, a bug on the window, or a lump of dough under my rolling pin, I didn't care. I wanted to *not* think about everything. At times, I wished I could flip my brain's switch to "Off."

God made me a deep thinker, which is both a blessing and a curse. Mix that up with my extreme sensitivity, emotional intelligence, and great understanding, and you've got yourself one seriously unique (aka weird) girl. You don't want to be a deep thinker when you have cancer, trust me. My own mind freaked me out on several occasions.

I found myself thinking, "Stop thinking!"

⸙

My mom talked with JY and Vicki, who had visited me during my second round in the hospital, via cell phone. They asked how to find the side entrance near the Cancer Center, so they could meet us for my clinic appointment in Santa Barbara. I interrupted their conversation.

"Just tell them to follow the bald people!" I bellowed.

Mom and I strolled into the Cancer Center's library. Whoa, there were a lot of books. TV crew members set up cameras, placed microphones, and ran wires just about everywhere. After shaking many hands and greeting the others, Mom took one chair while I took the one right next to it. Paula Lopez, our local newsperson, sat across the way. A man who called himself Rusty gave us little microphones to feed up and hook to our shirts. Then, it was lights, camera, and action.

I was being interviewed for The Children's Miracle Network Telethon that would air in May. Jaynie had pulled me aside one day and asked me if I would be interested in sharing "my story."

To be honest, I thought, "*What* story?" but agreed anyway.

⸙

I wanted to help those kids in the future who passed through Cottage Children's Hospital. As Paula eloquently recited questions, and I answered, I noticed that, hey, maybe I *did* have a story. But if, indeed, I did, I didn't really think that anyone would *want* to hear it.

The bright lighting, big camera, and multiple people watching made me feel slightly uneasy. It wasn't because of any sort of fear; heck, I could pull out twenty *fouettes* in front of them . . . *and* land each one. Seriously now, I really didn't think "my story" was special, and I almost felt as though I was complaining with my answers. But I was only telling the truth, the sad truth.

Post-interview we hightailed it up to the Peds clinic.

"Hey, why not stop in and pick up a quick bag of chemo while we're here?" I thought.

Nah . . . just joking. Unfortunately, it was mandatory. It was a long visit. Because I had passed out during my previous round, Nurse Pam made sure to tank me up with an extra large bag of fluids before sending me off. It took *forever* to drain into me, and I almost wished they would just give me a straw and stick it in the top, like a Capri Sun. But then again, I was a bad water drinker, and that was the whole reason I was being made into the world's first human water balloon in the first place.

Luckily, John, aka, JY, and Vicki were there to keep me company. It meant a lot to me to see their understanding and loving smiles across the room from the table I sprawled on. JY entertained me, and just about everyone else, as he sat at the plastic kiddy table in the corner. A coloring book was open in front of him, with an earthmover picture half-colored in with a pink crayon. After completing his coloring, he taped it up on the clinic wall, without any staff permission whatsoever.

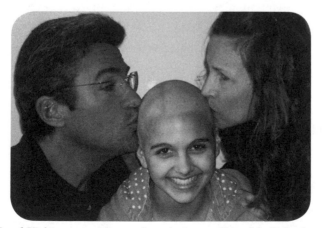

JY and Vicki return with more love during my Round 3 clinic chemo.

That guy cracks me up. He's like a grown-up big kid, in the sense that he plays, jokes, and enjoys life. I think we should all be kids. Not immature, just more carefree—not so serious. Yeah, life would be a lot more fun that way. So, as I observed JY's pink earthmover proudly displayed on the wall, I found myself free for a moment—giggling and entirely happy until I once again found myself home.

❧

"Jar," I read. "Hmm . . . Poppy, can you think of a four-letter synonym for 'jar'?"

Of course, I had one of my grandpa's witty comebacks thrown at me. Mom was out doing errands, so Poppy was on Melinda patrol. I'll tell you, about five minutes in with him, my stomach already hurt from laughing. Working to complete the morning crossword puzzle together, we conjured up all kinds of crazy things. We couldn't fill in *anything*, and I joked with Poppy, "Gee! Thanks for helping me!"

A session of giggles would follow. I didn't give a flying toot about the puzzle. It was the laughter that was priceless. And we were actually *good* at that!

❧

Cracking open my eyes, I observed the first morning light. It was a different morning. I had someone on my mind—my grandpop. Grandpop, or G-pop as I call him, is my grandpa who passed away the previous June. I am not sure why I awoke thinking about him, but I did. Imagining his gentle, soft smile that always graced his lips, I honored and acknowledged his strength and bravery. I pondered: "You know . . . he was my hero, *my* hero. He dealt with so much, yet the same calm, peaceful manner was always present in him. He was a beautiful person, and I love him beyond what words can describe."

I stared up at the high ceiling, wondering if he knew what was happening to me. Just milliseconds after that thought left my brain, I corrected myself. Of course he did. He was up there with God, probably sitting next to Him. I pictured G-pop, swooping down to look after me when I needed it and watching over me as I slept. Feeling a sense of serenity, I played the recorded G-pop tape in my head over and over, hearing his quiet, unique chuckle. And as I wrote this paragraph, I could've sworn he was with me in my room. I felt a presence . . . I sure hope it was him. Love you, G-pop.

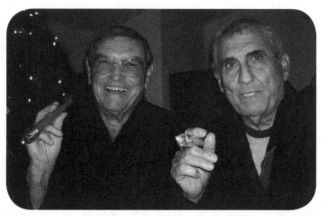

My two favorite grandpas, Poppy and G-pop, Christmas 2006.

Amalia, my home nurse, sped away with more of my blood to be tested. I felt *horrible*, and low blood counts were thought to be the cause. I even slept during the day, which is highly unusual for me. I don't believe in naps. Time ticked on, only heightening my suffering. I shut my eyes.

"Just go away," I thought.

A haunting, eerie pulse thumped *everywhere* in my body, and I mean everywhere. The deep, slow beat was so disturbing that I couldn't fall asleep, and I remained wide awake, my fright preventing me from peaceful rest. Although I *did* want to escape to dreamland, I was scared I wouldn't wake up. I didn't trust my body to fight for me while I slept. Like a drum, my head and heart pounded, as if they were trying to pump cement. I felt faint . . . slowly fading . . . slowly fading. My lungs expanded and contracted with my deep, therapeutic breaths. Sometimes they helped. Other times, they made me more light-headed.

Weakness overpowered me—a slight oxymoron, but oh so true. I thought about moving, but that was it; that's as far as I got. Examining Mom's pitch dark room, I took note of the time. 11:45. I wondered how much longer I could take it. Not able to fall asleep while I was so tense, I had to relax. But I was terrified to relax so much that my sleep would be permanent.

I'm not sure when, or how, but sleep eventually sucked me under. Strangely, I dreamed. Although I can't recall the actual dreams themselves, I sure do remember how I felt. I was sick—sick in my dreams. Feeling sick had become so common for me that it was *part* of me. I awoke distraught. Dreams are supposed to be just that . . . a *dream* . . . perfect, nice, whatever fancies your mind creates, but no, not me. There was no escaping being sick. I felt trapped, like I was taped in a cardboard box with no air holes. I was no longer at peace, even asleep.

My eyes caught sight of my reflection in the side mirror of our truck. I looked terrible. My image scared me. We whizzed down the 101 freeway toward Cottage Hospital. I had to do it. I had to get a transfusion. With Nicholas driving, Mom watched me from the backseat as I drifted closer and closer to unconsciousness. I'm sure it was one of the longest drives of her life; at last, we pulled up in front of the hospital. With one look, Mom knew I needed a wheelchair. Preparing to make the journey into its seat, I was thoroughly convinced that if I walked anywhere, I would die.

Invisible, thousand-pound weights were strapped to every cell in my body. The three of us loaded into the elevator, and Mom slapped the Floor 6 button, the adult floor. The Peds floor was entirely booked up—stuffed to the gills. Fortunately, Dr. Dan had called up to the Transfusion Suite on the adult floor, and a very accommodating nurse agreed to take me in—adopt me for the day. This lady was Nurse Jen, and she greeted us with enthusiasm as we entered.

Glancing around, I felt on top of the world. At nearly the highest point in the whole hospital, giant windows displayed the big, oncoming winter storm. It looked beautifully creepy. My vision adjusted back to inside, and I observed the small, connecting rooms. Three or four elderly people sat, casually reading magazines, while bags of blood pumped into them. It was a sight, nothing like I had imagined. It almost seemed like a cocktail party, but with blood. Everyone was laid-back and at ease—completely normal despite the IVs in their arms, administering the red stuff. The atmosphere was relaxed. Hmm, maybe it wouldn't be so scary. After all, at that point, I would have done almost anything to feel better.

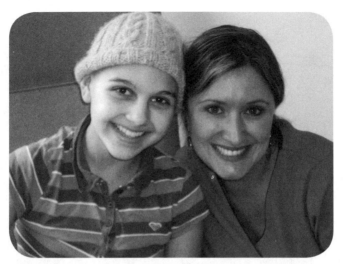

Nurse Jen adopts me for the day.

After chowing down my vegetarian tostada, I remember Nurse Jen teasing me about picking out the kidney beans. I filed a mental note to order it without them, if a next time came. Finally, after a lot of waiting, my blood . . . uh, well, *someone's* blood, arrived at the suite. O negative, baby.

Nurse Jen hooked me up, and I slid back in my huge, minty green armchair. It was really comfy. For some odd reason, I wasn't expecting to see the blood pumping toward me, because when "tomato juice," as Dr. Dan called it, began to seep out into the long tube, my heart did a funny skip. The long IV line ran out of my port, dragged on the ground, and finally rose to meet a close cousin of Ricco. It must have taken at least two minutes for the blood to finally reach me. I watched every inch of its journey along the tube, and the nearer it came, the more uneasy I felt. I wasn't scared of it, but I wanted my own body, with my own blood.

I felt like so much had been put into me that I barely *was* me anymore. I didn't want to be different, a mix of drugs, chemo, and a stranger's blood. Finally, it was within inches. It crept so slowly, it seemed, and at last it disappeared into my shirt, and into my chest. I still pictured its inward journey.

"Hmm . . . it's probably in my port now, and now, it's most likely . . . in my heart. And now, it's probably everywhere."

Gazillions of emotions tied up into a knot that sat at the bottom of my stomach. Anger, fear, confusion, relief, gratitude, frustration. I was experiencing it all. But before long, my emotions turned to thankfulness and hope. Within a couple of hours, visible signs that it was working were beginning to form. One thing I happily recall was the change in my vision. I could see better, clearer.

Colors were brighter, and it didn't take as long for me to look at something and process, "Oh, that's a spoon."

Breathing became easier because my cells then carried their own supply of oxygen. Nurse Jen checked my blood pressure what seemed like every five minutes. Gradually, she liked the numbers more and more. My heart was no longer a machine gun, pumping at a billion miles an hour, and for a little while, I had to get used to not hearing and feeling it anymore.

Another huge relief was my head. It didn't feel like a boulder anymore. It didn't thump and throb; it only sat innocently on my shoulders, like any good head does. Slowly, I could feel a tiny speck of strength returning to my limbs. Wow. I considered it a miracle—a full-blown miracle—an *Oprah Show*–worthy miracle. To go from where I had been to cracking jokes with Nurse Jen was amazing.

My punchy side emerged, and with my new blood working wonders, I grabbed my IV line and began to wrap it around my dome. Hooking it behind my ears, I saw others giggling at my blood headband. My increasing silliness peaked as I balanced a water bottle atop my head. Locating a straw, I laid it across the lid of the bottle . . . it stayed. I was convinced I could balance *anything* on my shiny, grippy *cabeza*.

Burning up the rest of the time chatting with Nurse Jen, I silently praised, thanked, and paid homage to all who donate blood. I know that when people go to those little blood drives, they claim it "Saves Lives," but seriously, now, here I am. They aren't lying.

I walked out, yes . . . *walked* out. Heck, I almost ran out, I was so happy. I was like a car after an oil change, running smoothly once again. I look back on this day with fond memories. And, oh yes, my enormous thanks to the amazingly generous Somebody with the O negative blood. You gave me an incredible gift—my *life*.

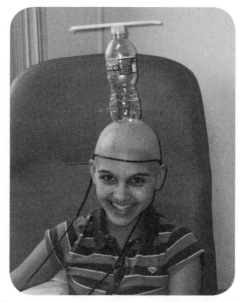

Me and my grippy *cabeza* in the Transfusion Suite.

"One word frees us of all the weight and pain of life:
That word is love." —Sophocles

FOURTEEN

TWO DAYS POST-TRANNY, or transfusion, I didn't need Dad to come in to stick me in the back of the arm anymore. We could discontinue the daily Neupogen shots. Another pleasant surprise came at dance. My energy—or, more so, lack of exhaustion—was very noticeable. Elated in the car on the way home from dance class that night, I shouted joyfully to Mom. I had done *everything*—yep, no sitting, resting, anything. It may not seem like much, but it meant *the world* to my spirit. It gave me amazing hope that I would, once again, do everything I once did—or more.

Mom pulled up to the curb to pick me up. As I tumbled into the car, she saw my face and knew something was wrong. I was never, ever, this way after dance class. Like a little kid, I was alright until she asked me if I was okay; then I began to cry. My language nearly incomprehensible, I explained that, in the upcoming recital, I wouldn't be able to dance in a ballet piece. That was what I had looked forward to. My light at the end of my dark tunnel was being on that stage, cherishing my passion while the hot stage lights glowed and the music thumped in my heart.

I was the only dancer enrolled in the Advanced Ballet class who wasn't part of the Youth Company. I hadn't been able to audition for the company because I was seriously ill at that time. The dance that they had begun to work on in class was a Youth Company dance, so there was little me, with my broken heart, plopped cross-legged in the corner watching everyone else dance their souls out.

Witnessing the Mama Bear expression across Mom's face, I was unsure of what plans of action she already had brewing. I saw that something was already in the works, though. There's no misinterpreting when she's determined.

Mom sent an email the very next day to my dance instructor, Ms. Cynthia. She received a phone call in return. There had been a communication lapse. Ms. Cynthia didn't realize Mom had signed me up—and paid for my dance classes—at the beginning of the semester, even though I wasn't able to attend at that time.

I would be allowed to perform in a ballet dance in the spring recital. The tears that rolled down my face weren't shed from sadness, but rather from joy. Hope. I had hope. One goal was set before me, and I was sure that I'd reach it. Excitement oozed out of my every pore, and I relaxed in Mom's bed that night, imagining myself floating and skimming across the auditorium stage. I entered sleep with a smile still present on my face. What a beautiful way to let your dreams put you to rest.

⁀

Like we had done nearly every single morning that we'd awakened together, my mom and I opened our eyes, just happening to be facing one another, at the exact same time. Must have been the silent wake-up call brain waves I was sending her . . . or she was sending me. As always, smiles shone on our "bubble faces," the term we use for the odd, swollen appearance of morning faces.

"Guess what?" I asked, stretching out my arms.

"What?" Mom replied.

"I had a dream last night that someone was trying to access my port, but I didn't have any numbing cream on."

All was silent, no reaction whatsoever. Mom wore a strange, blank stare.

"You know what?" she finally asked.

"What?" I answered, slightly puzzled.

"*I* had a dream last night that *I* had a port, and someone was trying to access it, but *I* didn't have any numbing cream on."

Whoa. Okay. I was thoroughly confused and disturbed, yet, at the same moment, I was thinking this was the most awesome thing I had ever heard of.

No way. I mean, really? What are the chances? We had the same *exact* dream, on the same *exact* night? Wow. Dream transfer. Mom and I were getting good, *really* good . . . ha, ha . . . *freaky* good. Staring at one another in astonishment, we determined that it was solid proof that we're twins born a generation apart.

The clue was, "Ballerina's attire."

Aha! I scribbled in "T-U-T-U" with my favorite pen.

The corresponding clue across was, "Restore to health."

Thinking for only a moment, I wrote "C-U-R-E" in giant, black letters. And then, it hit me. Tutu . . . cure. Cure . . . tutu. The cross the two words made suddenly hit me. It was beautiful—symbolic. These were the two things in life that I waited and yearned for, *healing* and *dance*. It was God delivering the morning paper to me.

At this point in time, things began looking up. I'm sure my mom still remembers the sight of me running (well, at least in my mind) out of dance and toward the car, waving a ballet costume order form wildly in my hand. Despite the extreme weakness of my muscles, my frequent dizziness and nausea, as well as, well, a lot of other junk, signs of improvement were becoming visible.

I began to attempt more "normal" activities. I wrote a school paper on radiation; I did my best pushing a rake around the yard; and I even completed my very first entire *pointe* class. I had been putting on my *pointe* shoes each night and struggling to execute a simple *relevé*, but I saw an increase in strength resulting from my diligence.

Also, I stretched. Before I got sick, I was able to do the splits on my left side and almost on my right. As I fell into a forward, left-legged split, I caught myself with my arms—almost there. Maybe I hadn't lost as much as I thought.

Another snippet of good news came when Mom stopped and looked at me, commenting, "Your cheeks are rosy!"

I had been paler than pale for months, but my face, at last, was blushed with the smallest, most discreet tint of pink. Mom told me she was starting to see "glimpses of health." I still felt horrible, and I still struggled and fought daily, but I decided to believe her. I trusted her.

Even though I was in my body, and knew how I felt, I thought, "Hey, maybe I at least *look* better."

⤚

Walking down the hospital halls, I was in awe that I had already been through, and *made it* through, three rounds. Just thinking about everything exhausted me and made me short of breath. I only became more light-headed as I sat in the tiny, clear box I called the Pope Mobile, performing my pulmonary function test. Having done one before my first round, I was already familiar with the demoralizing routine. The neon pink nose clip added giggles to the borderline hysterical process. I sat on a swivel chair, in my own personal telephone booth, my hands squishing the air out of my cheeks. Jamming my lips around a large tube, I repeated the series of three tests over and over.

"Suck in, hold, hold, hold, hold."

The technician on the speaker directed my every move.

"Hold, hold, hold."

Ugh. My lungs shriveled.

"Hold, hold, hold."

Oh my gosh. If chemo didn't kill me, this would.

"Hold! Okay, now blow! Blow! Blow!"

I blasted the air out of my lungs.

"As hard as you can! Blow! Blow!" Sandra commanded with enthusiasm.

My eyes bugged out, and I looked like an ape trying to whistle. I could've sworn I was breaking out in a sweat.

"Blow! Blow! Blow! Keep blowing!"

Ah! I screamed and laughed at the same time inside my head. It was painfully hysterical. I looked to Mom, who held back her laughter. Gee, thanks a lot. I probably set a *Guinness World Record* for sucking, holding, and blowing. I wanted my trophy. *Now.*

⤚

Once I had completed my lung workout for the day, I moved on to the next tests, an EKG and an echocardiogram. I was convinced that, after the pulmonary function test, they would discover that my heart had completely exploded. The room was dark, and the cool gel on my chest wasn't the greatest feeling in the world. The echo was a long process, and I gazed out the window at the trees. With my chest hurting from the pressure of the camera, which nearly caved in my diaphragm, I was relieved when the technician, Don, gave me an affirmative.

"Okay, we're done."

Phew. Now, I was moving on to the simple EKG. It took just minutes. The only discomfort was the coolness of the sticky squares they placed on me and, of course, ripping all of them off. As I peeled off the last sticky, lightning fast, I shuddered to think of a man with a disturbing, overly hairy chest getting an EKG. Yikes. I made sure the squares were all taken off and there were no stragglers. Twice, I had found sticky squares on me days after surgery. It was harder to rip them off the longer they stayed on me. I wonder who sells those little things. Hmm, I bet they make a lot of money. Ha, ha, maybe in college I'll major in sticky squares.

⌒

"Alright, here we go again," I thought, lying down in my hospital bed that was as starchy as a potato.

I had just forced down a horrible-tasting sandwich that I ordered for lunch, and it wasn't settling well. I'm sure it was actually delicious, but the mixture between drugs and anxiety temporarily stunned my taste buds.

My neighbor behind the curtain didn't help. She was, well . . . kind of . . . obnoxious. She was everywhere but her bed, and Jaynie had to keep telling her to get back in her room. To top it off, we had brought cookies that I baked for the nurses, and guess who wanted one? And another? And *another*? Anyway, I was extremely happy when Nurse Sue pulled aside the curtain, and a staff member changed the sheets on my ex-neighbor's newly vacated bed. I hopped into those freshly changed sheets on the bed next to the window, and relished another private suite.

I giggled as I saw the Cottage Hospital dry erase board on the wall in my room. Dr. Dan was on vacation, and under "Physician" I had sarcastically written, "On Vacation," "None," "Gee, thanks a lot," and my favorite, "He couldn't handle me."

But man, I understood why he needed a trip . . . I had been a tough case to solve—a hard safe to crack—a hard code to, uh, decode. I wanted to take a break from me too. I was jealous.

꩜

Thankfully, I wasn't entirely doctor-less. I had someone to look after me, and his name was Dr. Josh, a man from Stanford who not only acted and sounded like a doctor, he *looked* like a doctor. He was young, but his knowledge made him seem older. Dr. Josh had wide eyes and a quirky smile, and he shared with me that, ironically, he had battled Hodgkin lymphoma at age fifteen.

"Be careful," he warned. "One of the side effects of treatment is becoming an oncologist."

I laughed. Although I missed Dr. Dan a lot, having Dr. Josh mixed things up a little, freshened it up a bit—not that Dr. Dan was moldy or stale or anything.

꩜

My last CT scan had shown that I would, in fact, need radiation. An elderly man entered my hospital room and greeted me with a peaceful smile and sparkling eyes. It was my new radiologist, Dr. Weisenburger. No, not hamburger, not cheeseburger, not even veggie burger. Weisenburger. I distinctly remember thinking his tie was really, really cool. I think it had Bugs Bunny or someone like that printed on it. And that's pretty much what kept my focus as he discussed what the road ahead would bring. I tried to concentrate, I really did . . . but I was just so gosh darn tired. Not able to interpret a single word he said, I hoped that at least Mom was catching it in case he said something important. I was as attentive as a two-year-old . . . but I couldn't really help it.

My last round was the most enjoyable of the four. Many smiles and laughs helped keep me focused on the big picture, instead of minute by minute struggles. The medical staff and I poked fun at each other, now being closely bonded by my frequent appearances at the hospital.

One episode I can recall quite clearly. The morning sun awoke and rose over the majestic Santa Barbara Mountains. Shortly after, I saw Dr. Josh peeking in my door before entering swiftly and stopping abruptly.

"Good morning," he said meaningfully.

That was one thing about Dr. Josh. When he told you anything, you could tell that he was real, that he really meant it.

I stared back at that genuine look in his eyes, smiled, and mimicked, "Good morning."

Oh boy, I could tell it was coming. Vigilantly, I waited, watched, hesitated, until finally I got my cue.

"How are you doing?" he asked.

"Well . . . ," I muttered, wearing a suspicious smile that was probably quite blatant.

"I've noticed a little swelling in my hands," I confessed.

With a furrowed brow, Dr. Josh responded, "Well, okay, we'll take a look at them."

He came closer. My prey neared my bed covers, which had my hands completely concealed underneath. Closer . . . closer . . . closer. It was time. Casually, I slid my hands out, revealing my huge, white Mickey gloves that I had gotten at Disneyland. There was a millisecond of terror, and then, Dr. Josh broke into giggles. Like the plague, the laugh traveled around the room, from my nurse, to Mom, to me. I liked playing games. As far as I was concerned, it got way too monotonous, repetitive, boring, and degrading lying there for hours and hours on end. Dr. Josh even joined in on the fun, examining the ridiculous gloves and diagnosing imaginary problems.

"Hmm . . . yes. Aha. You have some moderate blanching happening," he concluded, referring to their snowy white color.

I felt so silly, but loved it. There's something cool and awesome about acting goofy and borderline stupid sometimes. It makes me feel like such a kid and like nothing else matters at that second, except laughing my guts out. Some people are afraid to act this way. Don't worry . . . God won't strike us with lightning if we have a good time . . . that's what He wants for us. One valuable lesson I've learned is to always be myself . . . no matter what other people think. Hey, if they don't like it—so what? I'm me, and although it sounds harsh, deal with it.

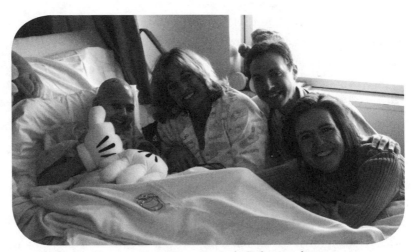

Gotcha! Nurse Pam, Dr. Josh, Robyn, and me.

The chemo and drugs were just beginning to loosen me up as Jaynie arrived with a small pack of glittery flower stickers. I grabbed them with excitement, and immediately began searching for the perfect spot to stick them. Hmm... let me see. The bed? No. My tray? No. Ricco? No. Hmm ... my head? Ha, ha, ha, ha, yes. Briskly peeling them off the paper, I arranged them evenly on my scalp. They stuck nicely.

Shortly after, the parade of therapy dogs began. Jaynie had done it again. My very first chemo of my fourth round began to drip as Ryder, the cute, soft-eyed chocolate Lab appeared bedside with a goofy grin. Of course, he wanted up ... and I wanted him up. With a soft pat on my sheets, his owner gave him the go ahead. I pet his soft ears and stared into his brown eyes. They matched his fur perfectly. I could see the innocence deep within them, the kind of carefree, happy-go-lucky innocence that I wanted in my life.

Just then, something caught those big, sweet eyes, something shiny. Uh-oh ... my stickers! Lunging for my shiny dome, he began frantically licking, trying to remove them, eat them, and play with them. Mom, and especially Ryder's owner, might have been expecting a slight freak out, but instead, I was laughing so hard that people outside probably thought the chemo was making me insane. I'm actually very much in awe that no one hucked me in the loony bin through all of this. I was like a clown: giggling, goofy, and silly on the outside, but pained and scared on the inside. Not to be stereotypical or anything, but clowns seem

like pretty disturbed people . . . that must be why they decide to become clowns.
I felt like a clown—Chemo the Clown.

It was a Thursday night . . . not that it mattered or anything. I never knew
what day it was, or what time it was. I barely knew what month it was. Oh,
March . . . right. Mondays had become Wednesdays, Fridays, and Sundays—
anything *but* Mondays. The same goes for all of the other days. But I remember
this Thursday vividly.

The piano keys felt cool as my fingertips brushed them. The bench on which
I sat creaked with my shifting weight. Ricco stood nearby; his constant pumping sound was drowned out by the melody each piano key gave birth to. With
smiles of pure joy, and eyelashes as dams to hold back their oncoming tears,
many of the nurses who I love dearly watched and listened. We sat on the adult
floor, the big windows displaying the transformation of day into night.

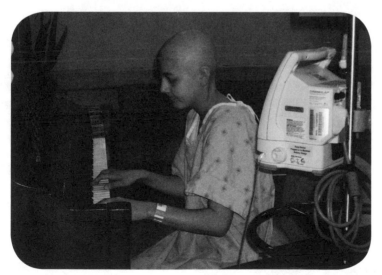

Playing "Can't Help Falling in Love with You" for my nurses.

I played what I knew: the first song that came, not to my mind, but to my
heart. "Can't Help Falling in Love with You" was the only song that I was so

familiar with that my hands just went, just played it. I couldn't remember anything else because of my half-dead, chemo brain. To be honest, I didn't even remember the song that I played, but I only had to know where to start, and everything would go from there. I didn't know when to hit B, C, or F—I just found myself playing the right keys. Some may call it muscle memory. Personally, I call it spirit memory. I only messed up once or twice . . . when I thought too much.

⌒

I wanted a party . . . a killer party . . . one of those parties that you remember for a long, long time afterward. I wanted to celebrate my last day of chemo in the hospital and, also, wanted to thank the staff for everything they'd done for me. Mentioning it to my mom, I knew there was no way she would refuse.

I started preparing, making sashes, a game, and a poster that read "*Melinda's Last Chemo, Thank You, and Dance Party.*"

I wrote the time, and my room number, in sloppy letters beneath and had Mom tape it up outside my door. The game I created was a Melinda Original— Pin the Bag of Chemo on the Mass. Carefully drawing intricate, little bags of chemo, I made each one perfectly. It's something you only do if you literally have all the time in the world. Lying in the hospital can give a person a serious case of OCD.

Next in my hospital art studio was the creation of The Giant Card. It was for Dr. Josh, and it was a 3-foot × 5-foot masterpiece, if I might say so myself. I couldn't merely make him a normal card—I wasn't normal.

Coloring the huge block letters spelling out, "Thank You, Dr. Josh," I told Mom, "I want to give him something he has to lug around."

I taped and glued just about everything to it. Examination gloves, medicine cups, sterile wipes, and those sticks they use to squish your tongue down were all adorned with flashy, silvery glitter.

My lunch arrived right in the middle of my project. I felt I was far too busy to eat, but quickly observed my food options. Opening my bowl of soup, I found an unexpected item floating amid its brothy liquid. Nurse Nancy and Nurse

Gail surprised me—with a plastic fly swimming in my soup. Laughing, I turned to them, and their sneaky expressions changed to smiles. Ah . . . I loved it. Thank God I didn't get boring nurses. I would have died, not of cancer but of boredom. We all decided that I should tape the fly on Dr. Josh's card, and once it was securely fastened, I observed my work. Beautiful. He was going to love it.

It was a busy day. Besides my speedy preparations for the party, a man named Jorge stopped by to film me for my Children's Miracle Network vignette. He was an extremely tender man, with a smile that stretched so wide I could've sworn his lips would snap like a rubber band. Boing! With his face hidden behind his large camera, he interviewed me, asking about the *Beads of Courage* strung around my neck. This is also when Nurse Cyndi entered with my last bag of chemo I would receive in the hospital.

A strange tingle tickled my insides as I told myself, "Almost there . . . almost there."

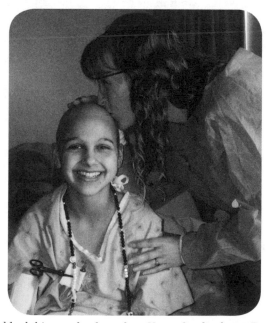

A good luck kiss on the dome from Nurse Cyndi, chemo Round 4.

A saline flush was hooked to my IV line, like two pipes fitting together. Hmm, now that I think of it, that's all they really were—pipes. And those pipes fed into my pipes, my chemo-clogged pipes.

When I looked at Nurse Cyndi, I clearly remember asking her, "Can I flush myself?"

She smiled, gently handing the saline to me, and replied, "Sure."

Grabbing the small, plastic tube, I hesitated for a second. Wow. I had always braced against the discomfort induced by others, but had never really created my own discomfort. I was fascinated, disturbed, invigorated, and uneasy. Steadily pushing it, the normal, salty, somewhat bitter taste appeared in the back of my throat. For some reason, I expected that when I did it, that wouldn't happen, it wouldn't feel that way.

A strange combination of emotions blended inside of me. Distraction chased them away as Jorge continued to record me. Slightly confused, I wasn't sure if I was Children's Miracle Network material. I didn't think I was sick enough or looked that in need. Did I really look *that* bad? Should I act happy or like I was dying? What did they want from me? Whoa. It was getting way too complicated. I just decided to be myself, my joyful, cheerful self.

Before my video session, Mom mentioned to Jorge that I was having a party later on, and she invited him to come and tape some footage. She also told him I would be getting my last chemo later that morning, and he could tape then if he wished to. Jorge chose the chemo taping; they wanted tear-jerking, heart-wrenching video.

Boy was he surprised when he walked in to see smiling, gleeful Melinda. I wasn't about to put on a false front for the camera. This was who I was. I don't mean to sound insensitive, but take it or leave it. Showing the world exactly what I was about, I knew that I wasn't a very good Children's Miracle Network child. I was too happy, too smiley, too full of life.

My grin screamed, "Hey! This is me! Melinda! And my specialty is having a good time when it's freakin' impossible!"

Long story short, Jorge packed up his camera and was out the door promising, "I'll be back for the party."

My guests would be arriving shortly. I took one last glance at my room. Everything was perfect. The game hung on the opposite wall; the pink sashes were lined up nicely; the cookies were out; and Ricco was dressed for the occasion, with crepe paper and a balloon adorning him. I even got spruced up, feeling like a million bucks with a pink balloon taped to the top of my head.

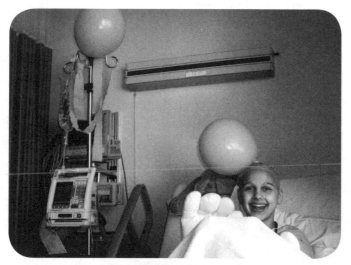

Ricco and I ready to party!

Asking Mom what time it was, I anxiously, and excitedly, awaited their momentary arrival. Just then, I heard noise in the hall: not hospital noise, *happy* noise. Suddenly, I heard their loud chants nearing my room. I finally recognized what the group was chanting.

"No more che-mo! No more che-mo!"

Oh my gosh. It was them. Within seconds, the mass of familiar faces took my room by storm. As they continued to chant, I noticed their toy blowers, maracas, and crowns.

Nurse Pam broke free from the crowd and came over to me. My expression displayed shock, surprise, and excitement as she plopped a giant gift bag on my bed and placed a tall, plastic crown atop my head. I felt like a princess. They had brought the party to me, and I sat there in a state of total and complete disbelief at how much love poured out of their hearts and flowed into mine. The best part was I didn't even need an IV to receive the love they gave me. Entirely touched and in awe, I quickly switched gears . . . it was time to have some *fun*. I turned on the party music, and it began to play quietly on the hospital's sad excuse for a sound system. It was the *Alvin and the Chipmunks* soundtrack.

Originally, I had wanted to play "The Hamster Dance" song, but was appalled to discover, during my party preparations, that it had been accidentally erased from my iPod. I broke down crying—I'm not sure why. As soon as one teardrop hit my pillow, Mom had taken off in the car to search out "The Hamster Dance" CD, or my next choice, "Alvin and the Chipmunks," while I slept to rest up for my party. There was no way Mom would let anything ruin my party plans.

"Funky Town" was cranked up to the highest volume as I bounced up and down. The Mickey gloves that never left my hands were high in the air.

Everyone broke out in hysterics as Nurse Pam got down with her bad self, and the group chanted, "Go Pam! Go Pam!"

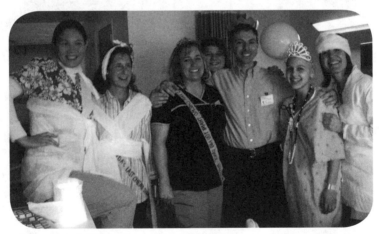

Zippy, Jaynie, Nurse Pam, Nanci, Dr, Josh, me, and Robyn during my
Last Hospital Chemo Party.

The party only heated up from there. After a rousing game of Pin the Bag of Chemo on the Mass, we had another fun activity I proudly invented myself. Toilet paper outfits. I watched as Jaynie was wrapped up like King Tut, with even a headband made out of the white paper. Robyn, the social worker from the clinic, was a good sport as she was twisted around and around to complete her toilet paper shirt. And the clinical trial specialist from the clinic, Zippy, also wore a unique getup. I gave Dr. Josh his card.

It was a total surprise to him, and if his expression could talk, it would have said, "Wow, you shouldn't have."

He was probably already contemplating how to get it into his car. Unfortunately, Dr. Josh had to leave the party early, so I thanked him for everything and watched as he disappeared out the door, his giant card securely tucked under his arm. I've emailed Dr. Josh a few times since then, and he confessed to me that he still couldn't figure out how to hang it up in his office. How about now, Dr. Josh? Any luck?

Munching cookies and swaying to the music, everyone looked like they were having a great time. It must have sounded like a pretty killer party too, because a strange girl I didn't recognize wandered in, her eyes glued to the large platter of chocolate chip and Snickerdoodle cookies. She must have been the sister of another patient on the Peds floor, and it wasn't until post-party that I heard the gut-busting story that had happened with her. Apparently, within minutes of crashing my party, the little girl became whiny.

"I want a party!" she complained, with jealousy, to Jaynie, who happened to be standing nearby.

Jaynie's eyes grew wide, and a sort of odd smile formed as she paused. Then, gazing down at the girl, she spoke truthfully.

"Well, if *you* get cancer one day, you can have a party too!"

I'm pretty sure the girl had no comeback.

Leading a parade down the short halls of Peds, I waved to Jorge, who captured it all on film. Jaynie marched behind me, pulling Ricco and holding the back of my gown closed. Man, that Jaynie . . . she's always covering by butt . . . literally. All of my friends walked and cheered behind me. It was a beautiful moment.

I remembered back to the hundreds of times where I would just pick a spot and stare, for hours on end, concentrating on pushing through each second individually. I wondered how I made it through those moments, and then it came to me. I didn't give myself any other choice. There I was, *walking*, yes, walking down the halls, celebrating my first victory, my first checkpoint. I was well aware of the visible and hidden obstacles to come, but only wanted to rejoice in what I could at the time. The way I see life is a series of tiny triumphs. Eventually, they all piece together to form our life. And by acknowledging and celebrating each step along the way, we get to the end and treasure each joyful moment that we came upon.

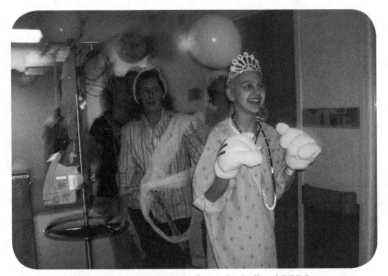

The celebratory parade down the halls of PEDS.

"But by the grace of God I am what I am. His grace which was bestowed upon me was not futile, but I worked more than all of them; yet not I, but the grace of God which was within me."
—World English Bible, I Corinthians 15:10

FIFTEEN

A SMALL VICTORY ensued four days after I returned home. I was out of my stinky PJ's and into real clothes, uh . . . well, actually, sweats. Close enough, to me. It was the same thing, only even more tiring the fourth time around. I ingested almost more pills than food, my legs killed me from the Vincristine, and my daily shots were getting *really* old. My dad and I became increasingly irritable with one another, although in a playful manner.

After giving him a hard time, he would reply, "Alright! Bend over! It's going in the butt this time!"

Amalia came, and as I expected, my blood counts were low. After four rounds of chemo, I wasn't really sure how I even had *any* blood cells left. With my head thumping, my vision a blur, and my heart racing a million miles an hour, I recognized all of the eerie, disturbing symptoms.

My Great-Uncle Johnny passed away, and a solemn, somber feeling in the house put a damper on my mood. It was one of those "what *now*?" days. But my dampened spirit, as well as my pack of Kleenex, was gracefully lifted on March 12, 2008.

Mom and I sat in the very, very back row, on the very end of the aisle, in the Marion Theater. Beautiful music hummed, filling the huge area with a sweet tone. I was afraid of the combination of my low blood counts and the crowd of germs seated in the rows of chairs below. But I wouldn't have missed this for anything.

We were here to watch a dance, dedicated to me by my previous dance instructor, Ms. Shelagh. Gorgeous. Peaceful. Calming. These are the words that come to mind when trying to describe it. Of course, it was ballet, and it wasn't until halfway through the dance that I realized that my mom was crying too. Our tissues were crushed balls in our palms, and our hands squeezed one another tightly. I felt love—nothing but love.

The twelfth of March got better and better. I thanked God as I took a swig of milk to choke down my very last prednisone—ever. What might be judged as a small victory to some was like winning a Nobel Prize to me. Waiting for the bitter taste to diminish, I looked forward to when I could truly relish my accomplishment.

Just one more time . . . one last time of that inhumane poison being injected into me. It was March 13, 2008, my very last chemo day at the clinic. A bittersweet sensation clung to me, like lint on a wool sweater. I was in a celebration mode, yet a defensive and battling mode. The reality that I *did* actually have to get chemo that day finally sunk in and dwarfed my excitement.

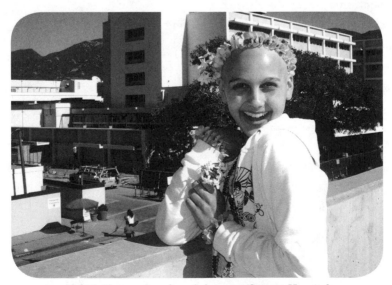

Aloha! My very last day of chemo at Cottage Hospital.

But my smiling face, along with the plastic lei on my head with matching wristbands, masked any disappointment. I guess I kind of wanted it to be like the last day of the school year, where all you do is watch movies, and you don't actually do any schoolwork. Yep, that's what I was hoping for.

⁓

The elevator doors slid open, and I felt like I nearly walked straight into the tall man standing inside. Glancing up, I saw it was Dr. Pickert. Oh my gosh, this was freakin' awkward. I wanted a different elevator. Just then, the doors slid closed . . . too late. Leaning on the wall opposite him, I don't recall making immediate eye contact, but I could *feel* him looking at me. The elevator ascended, and I watched each floor indicator light up as we passed. The silence was so dense you could've cut it with a knife. I had a silent conversation with myself.

"Does he remember me? I'm not sure. Should I say something? Is he trying to avoid me? I don't think so, but if he is, that's pretty funny, and you *should* say something. What's that weird smell? Hmm, it's either BO or mashed potatoes. Wait. Yep—definitely mashed potatoes."

The longest elevator ride of my life sped up as I began to hear a voice other than my own. Dr. Pickert spoke. He asked me something like whether he had done a procedure on me. Smiling sweetly, I replied that yes, he had inserted my PICC line in the PICU. We reached our destination, and the doors parted.

"Weren't you the one with the difficult awakening?" he inquired, as he prepared to exit.

I gave him an affirmative, and so did Mom.

After we said good-bye, and Dr. Pickert was well away from the elevator, I joked, "I'll show *you* a difficult awakening!"

Mom and I broke into a roar of laughter. The truth was, I had no hard feelings toward Dr. Pickert, but I was just using our situation to produce a little humor. I found our awkward relationship hysterical and couldn't help but do some harmless teasing.

Putting on my best disgusted, threatening expression, and using my perfected New York dialect, I huffed, "Get outta here, ya Ketamine pusha!"

⁓

It seemed like the same old shebang as my very last ml of chemo traveled down my IV tube, into the world of Melinda or, more so, my own personal microscopic cancer war zone. The only thing that differed was the crown and sash Nurse Pam wore, which she had saved from my party, and the tinge of anxiety in the air.

Dr. Kelts, the pediatric gastroenterologist down the hall, let me listen to "Dancing Queen" on his iPod, and Jaynie stopped by with Jorge's DVD of my party. I thought it was sweet of Jorge to do that for me, and I knew that as years and years went on, that DVD would mean more and more. Staring at the chemo-eyed picture of me on the disk, I began to feel the effects of my present chemo. Many congratulations echoed down the hall after me as I left the clinic, excited and triumphant, yet knowing my fight was not over.

❧

The world was fuzzy and dark—on account of my eyelids being barely a quarter of the way opened. Mom and I drove past the Blueberry Farm, and I saw it fade to black as my eyes slammed shut. Exhaustion does not begin to describe the sheer magnitude of my fatigue. I felt I was going to die of tiredness . . . I really did. Everything felt so faint, so weak, so nonexistent.

As we finally reached home, the bump going up our driveway forced me into a somewhat alert consciousness. I dragged myself inside and, with Mom's help, climbed into bed. Unable to get even remotely comfy, I cried, and cried, and cried. Staring at the ballet *barre* mounted on the opposite wall, I unintentionally acknowledged exactly how much I was suffering, and how much physical trauma was haunting my body. It was not good when I thought of how sick I was. Torture, that's how I describe that evening. It was torture. I had considered it a special day . . . but for just a short time.

❧

Looking down at the majority of my eyelashes clumped in my washcloth, shock, and a sort of sick amusement, triggered my strange reaction. It was one of those moments where your brain knows that something is wrong with the picture you're looking at, and you feel really dumb because you can't quite figure it out. I did, finally, grasp that if they were down there, then they certainly weren't *up* there anymore. It was a blonde moment. No wait, I didn't have any hair, so I'm off the hook. The last of the bodily hair to go were my eyebrows. I specifically remember appearing in the kitchen one foggy March morning in my long, hot pink robe.

Nicholas sat at the table and, upon looking at me, questioned, "Mushy! Where are your eyebrows?"

Now, how was I supposed to answer that?

"They're on a one-way cruise to Mexico?"

I honestly don't know what I was on, but I was in one of the silliest moods of my life. Fresh out of my bath, I was feeling "bald and proud," as I began to rub my head.

"Mom," I called. "You know how I was Ben before?" I asked with a crooked, goofy smile.

"Well, now I'm Phil!" I shouted spontaneously. "Phil Collins!"

Collapsed in the middle of the hall, Mom and I gasped for breath as deep, deep laughter made tears come out of our eyes. I have never, ever laughed that hard. I was at the point where I could literally have a cardiac arrest. And we could *not stop*. The image of the bald singing star was ingrained in my mind. It was so funny.

To send it really over the edge, I began to sing Phil Collins's *Tarzan* song, "Strangers Like Me." My horrible voice mixed with my uncontrollable laughing, which made it even *funnier*. It took us nearly a half hour to fully recover. My stomach killed me. I had nearly wet my pants several times. My head hurt, and I was exhausted. Ah . . . it was great. To top off what already topped things off, as Mom went to take her shower, post-laugh-fest, she flipped on the radio. Who greeted her with a song? Yep, it was my buddy, Phil.

☞

I'm aware of the mass quantity of times I've already stated this, but I was so sick of being sick that it made me even sicker. And then, I became sick of being sick of being sick. It was another phase of frustration and lack of patience, but luckily, I managed to find little things to do while slamming around the house.

One morning, I excavated every single beanie and hat that I owned and gave Mom a fashion show, and one night, we watched *The Bee Movie*. One day I tried on all of my wigs, including stuffed animal wigs, and one day Mom and I took a trip up to San Luis Obispo, about half an hour north of us. After using the Barnes & Noble gift card I received from my loving second cousins, Jim, Sissy, Jenna, and Alex, Mom and I cooled off with a Jamba Juice.

Yes, it was a warm day, pretty much the first time I strutted my bald stuff in public. Having always worn a hat or something, I felt the glares as I walked through crowds completely uncovered. It felt good and refreshing to let it all hang out. My main concern was that I didn't want to frighten people, but I soon realized that a note of surprise in folk's reactions was inevitable.

Waiting for our smoothies, a cute baby, snuggled in a stroller, caught my attention. Our eyes met, and as I smiled at the little one, the baby stared back in horror. "Baby" knew there was something wrong with me and was entranced by my shiny dome. The staring contest continued, and I began giggling with amusement. Fascination, shock, confusion, and terror were all painted across the baby's chubby-cheeked face. Mom and I laughed for hours afterward, and my assumption was that the little guy thought I was none other than a giant baby! It was, indeed, true to a certain extent. My mommy helped bathe me, she walked with me, she brought me food, and a diaper would have come in handy on one particular occasion. Sighing and laughing in a whiny tone, I felt like a giant baby. And oh yeah . . . I guess I was bald.

⌒

"Crud. That darn Bleomycin!" I thought as I gargled vigorously with a solution of warm water and salt.

My mouth sores hurt like the dickens and were caused by one of my five types of chemo, Bleomycin. The painful sores lined the inside of my mouth and made eating entirely un-enjoyable. I took comfort in knowing that it was the last time . . . the *very* last time I would have to deal with it.

Bleomycin is also the chemo that can mess with your lungs. Dr. Dan firmly told me that if I ever smoked after receiving Bleomycin, my lungs would "turn to cement." Ewwwww. That didn't sound too exciting. I joked with Mom, saying that at least I would have an excuse in high school next year not to cave in to peer pressure. I had my invisible script ready.

"Oh no, I can't man. I did some gnarly Bleomycin back in the day."

I was pretty sure it would work.

Amalia swooped in to draw labs and was gone in a flash. My port was a little sore from being accessed as I trudged tiredly about the house.

"I'm going to dance," I told Mom, who looked doubtfully back at me from her desk chair.

"I am," I stated confidently. "I'm going to dance."

Stubbornness in that area was something I was becoming known for.

Usually, when I made this statement, it translated to, "I really wish I could go to dance, but I'm not feeling well enough."

That day, though, I convinced Mom, and we sailed off to class. I emerged feeling better than when I had gone in and was on an incredible dance high that put me in a unique mood. Post-bath that night, I somehow got on the subject of Phil Collins once again.

Looking truthfully and honestly at Mom, I giggled, "I need a recording studio!" before breaking into another *Tarzan* song.

The after-dance fatigue usually hit me the next day. Slumping in my chair at the breakfast table, I asked Mom if Dr. Dan was still on vacation.

"I don't know. We haven't heard from him," she told me.

A mixture of drugs, tiredness, and "morning Melinda" influenced my sarcastic answer.

"Do I even *have* an oncologist anymore?" I asked.

"Look!" I shouted, whipping off my rainbow beanie and pointing at my dome.

"I *need* an oncologist!"

Once again, I provided the laugh for the day. My life was like a rubber band ball, or the world's largest chewing gum wad. With each new band or glob added, the weight of it all began to get heavier and more cumbersome. Each rubber band, or stick of gum, was an individual event I had gone through, but stepping back and looking at it all together was exhausting to a whole new degree. This is the way I felt. Shortness of breath was commonplace for me, and Mom described that I was "walking like I was in my golden years." Gee, thanks Mom.

⌒

"Alright, we'll see you then," Mom answered before hanging up the phone.

She told me that I wouldn't have Amalia today, but Joyce, another home health nurse. That instant, something hit the bottom of my stomach like a backhoe dumping dirt, and I retrieved the EMLA cream, to begin the gob-on session. An abnormal nervousness mounted as the doorbell rang.

Joyce entered, piled all of her gear here and there, and instructed me to lie down. While prepping a saline flush, it somehow squirted out, getting one of my favorite shirts wet and giving me a pre-bath bath. I lifted my shirt and looked away, thinking about how nice it would feel once it was all over.

Giant, man hands poked at my chest, and grabbing my port like a doorknob, she twisted it so roughly it made me grind my teeth in pain. Mom could see the tension throughout my body, my face that displayed my extreme discomfort, and the tight grasp with which I clung to the bedsheets. Uh-oh, here came the needle. Swallowing hard, I took a deep breath as the pressure seemed to crush me. Suddenly, I heard one of the most disturbing sounds of my life.

"Pop!"

Oh my gosh. What the $*@ did she hit?! Then she said something that only made it more of a nightmare, that turned it into the blood test from hell.

"Oops," she chuckled. "I think I missed it."

Yeah, you think? I couldn't believe how much my situation stunk. Helplessly pinned down, there was nothing to do but push through. Thankfully, with some major praying and finger crossing, the second time made it in. Dumbfounded and pissed, I remained there with my mouth sealed closed until it was over. On her way out the door, I found forgiving and respectful Melinda.

I uttered, "Thank you," as Joyce left.

And what did I hear called back at me?

"I know you don't really mean that!"

Ugh. It was hopeless. Why did I even try?

⌒

I refused to lie in the hospital bed, and when my lunch arrived, the smell nearly made me gag. I couldn't look at it. My first bag of blood drained into me; I was once again back in Peds, like a weird déjà vu. My blood test did not lie. I needed another tranny.

A headband with bunny ears was fastened on my dome, and a basket of candy-filled eggs had been dropped off at the nurses' station. Easter was the next day, and I gave a bright, colorful egg to Jake and to Aliyah, Dr. Dan's adorable, wide-eyed children. I didn't like being back there . . . it was depressing. Babies cried, kids moaned, and nurses were rushing everywhere.

Just outside my door, a small girl was motionless on a stretcher. My heart ached for her. I tried to ignore the cries of pain from my roommate as the nurse injected her with insulin. But what really ripped my soul out was when I saw a nurse walk by in her full, blue protective wear. Wow, she was going to give chemo to some poor child. I almost began to cry, but I had to disconnect for fear of having a breakdown. I couldn't help but wonder who it was, what they had, and how long they'd been fighting. That night was my release of emotions. I cried so hard, I nearly choked on my own tears. I felt those kids' pain . . . more than anyone knows.

Easter morning came, and as I looked outside, the absolutely gorgeous day God made reminded me exactly what Easter is all about. Our pool felt cool and refreshing on my feet. A smile pasted itself across my face. It was the very first time I had gone swimming in nearly a year. To me, this was a huge step toward "normal." Later in the day we went to my Grandma and Poppy's house, the place of gathering for our Easter feast, and I brought along many goodies I had cooked at home. It was a nice day, filled with many laughs. Happiness poured out of me—I was glad to have the previous day behind me.

Ba-bump! We drove into our local Chevron station to fill up before the drive to Santa Barbara. A CT scan was scheduled, and thoughts trickled out of my brain. I watched the squeegee slide back and forth as Mom cleaned our spring-time-bug-splattered windshield. Just then, I saw a stranger approach Mom. The woman wore a pleasant grin, and before I knew it, they were both nearing my window. A wave of confusion and puzzlement surfaced within me, and I opened the car door, slowly, to see what was going on.

I thought she might be an old friend that my chemo-ed-out brain could not locate in the memory banks, but found that I was mistaken when Mom surprised me by saying, "This nice woman wants to pray for you."

"What is your name?" the lady asked me.

"Melinda," I replied with uncertainty.

"Melinda," she repeated, her voice seeming unnaturally sweet and harmonic.

"God has told me to pray for you. Could I do that?"

Numb, I felt completely numb. My body, my mind, and my spirit—they were all entirely numb. Agreeing, I got a sudden chill, as she reached out and took my hand. This was unreal—*so* not happening. Her grasp was strong, loving, and comforting. It possessed the warmth that radiated throughout my body. And then, sitting in our truck at the Chevron station, holding a complete stranger's hand . . . I heard one of the most beautiful prayers of my life.

Awe and speechlessness formed a lump in my throat that grew with each of her tender, holy words. A sense of happiness, hope, and peace made me feel as though my soul was fulfilled—rejuvenated. Bursting from the inside out, I felt my spirit swell with love, gratitude, security, and emotions that are far too complex for the feeble human mind to intellectually understand. As with many, many things, I do not remember the words . . . but only the feeling.

At that moment, I felt closer to God than ever before. He was there . . . inside of me, inside of the woman, and all around us. He was the love that we were all experiencing at that very moment.

And with an, "Amen," I opened my eyes back to the "real" world and rediscovered where I was, and what was going on.

I had so much to say to her, but was stuck searching through the earthly dictionary to find something good enough. We got her name, Diana. God was working through Diana that day to speak to me, and she let God use her to truly touch my life.

⌒

With tears still clumped in our eyes, Mom and I began our journey down the freeway. Within minutes, I exploded into a gut-splitting laugh.

"What?!" my shocked mom asked.

Not able to find a breath to speak, I pointed to the windshield. Mom's half was spotless . . . mine was yellow, with wings, abdomens, and other undeterminable bug parts. Having cried once already, the tears flowed once more out of laughter.

"The most wasted day is that in which we have not laughed."
—Chamfort

SIXTEEN

CNN, LARRY KING, or one of those news shows flashed on the TV screen as I stared mindlessly at it. Mom read the paper in the chair next to me. We were at our local Marion Medical Center, waiting for my chest X-ray. Pretty bored, I caught sight of a little girl and her mother waiting near us. She was no more than three, and upon glancing at me, she began to stare with a frightened look. I chuckled. Here goes the giant baby stuff again. Waving at her, I watched as she ran back to her mother.

Tugging at her mom's pants, she exclaimed, "Look! Look!"

Her tiny finger pointed at me. Amusement extinguished any of my remaining boredom. Suddenly, my ears caught what my mind couldn't quite believe.

"It's a baby!" she shouted.

The girl's mother wore a horrified, apologetic look as my mom and I snorted and giggled.

Just when I thought it couldn't get any funnier, the toddler yelled, "*Big baby!*"

Her mom grabbed her, working frantically to hush her say-it-like-it-is child. I was the farthest thing from hurt.

"Well," I thought, "this confirms it. I *am* a giant baby!"

Looking to my mom in hysterics, I saw her face buried and hidden behind her newspaper. Ah . . . life is entertaining, one's own personal comedy show.

❧

By the end of March, only a few eyelashes still clung to my eyelids, and my eyebrows were becoming sparser with each new day. No longer did I have to fear the dreaded uni-brow. My energy was very low, but I somehow still found a speck to dance with. I was tired of the lifestyle of lying in bed, watching *Sponge-Bob* and eating ice cream—*it was so not me.*

❧

The second day of April was my first radiology appointment. Holding deathly still, I watched my radiologists, Kym and Sylvia, hovering over the CT scanner. With duo Sharpies, they marked the "field of radiation."

"What are you doing? Playing tic-tac-toe on me?" I joked.

Flashing their sweet smiles, I could see that they knew I was going to be a different one. After a brief meeting with Dr. Weisenburger, our day at Cottage Hospital came to a closing. Mom and I had wondered how Dr. Dan knew it was time for radiation, and that no more chemo was needed.

He always had concise, confident answers, and simply told us, "Statistics."

❧

I made Mom push the cart as we strolled through Vons. The last thing I wanted to do was touch that germ-infested handle. Errands, at that time, were fun for me. They were a "normal person" kind of thing, where I could be doing something with my mom and getting out of the house a little. Pulling into the checkout line, the lady behind the counter smiled at me. As we paid, she softly asked me what my name was.

I told her my name, and as we departed, she comforted me by saying, "I'm going to keep you in my prayers."

This was Susan, who has been praying for me ever since. Not a time goes by when we see her at Vons that she doesn't ask how I'm doing. My appreciation is overflowing into her lap.

❧

Mom read out of my science book as I sat leaning against the sliding glass door, listening intently. Learning was so cool, and I expressed a whole new excitement and appreciation for soaking up new things, "because I could." Brain lapses and repetitive reading were common, but I was simply happy to be able to think at all. On the subject of school, Mom and I attended the Freshman Orientation Night at Nipomo High School early in April. Yep, that's right. I was going to be "Freshmeat" . . . yikes.

Not too long post-chemo, my hair began germinating once again. What I did not expect was to feel so itchy . . . *everywhere*. Apparently, it was not just growing back on my head; I had lost it over my *entire body*. Lotion only provided temporary relief. It was my hair follicles reawakening. I felt like a giant bug bite. However, I avoided scratching for fear of disturbing the growth of the delicate fuzz.

After a beautiful day in the pool, Mom informed me that the water created bubbles on my tiny hairs. Another hair comment came when Nicholas helped me apply sunscreen.

"Mushy!" he shouted enthusiastically, "You have fuzzies!"

Even the girls at dance wanted to pet my fuzz.

We became anxious, waiting for the start of radiation. I wanted to be done—with it *all*. Luckily, I had some distractions. One was the Teddy Bear Cancer Foundation Family Fun Day. Our entire family drove out to Rancho Oso, in the Santa Barbara Mountains, for good food, miniature golf, a piñata, tennis, horseback rides, and an all-around great time.

I learned to rope, although I wasn't very good at it. But what really was the highlight of that day for me was seeing the other kids. They were all having such a good time and looked so happy. Many were bald, some had giant scars or were in a wheelchair, but the carefree expressions plastered on their faces touched me. And, wait, I guess I was one of those kids too, wanting just one day to *be a kid*.

"How are you feeling?" Mom asked me as we headed for, yep, you guessed it, Cottage Hospital.

"Pretty good," I dishonestly replied.

That's what I always said, just like my grand-pop. My dad told me that even if he was lying there in the ICU, fighting for his life, that would be his answer. I must have inherited that ability to subtly lie to put others at ease. My anxiety made it so I could not sit still, nor get comfortable whatsoever. A restlessness and impatience ticked like a bomb inside me. Not providing any assistance in the matter was the Tom Petty CD I had given Mom for her birthday playing in the background.

"The waiting is the hardest part . . . ," he sang.

Ugh. Don't remind me. I was overwhelmed with life.

Turning to Mom, I complained, "I hate having a condition."

More pre-radiation pictures, measurements, and blood tests took place. This time, the technicians drew on me with red Sharpies before placing stickers where they were needed. Supplied with nothing but a mound of alcohol pads to scrub off the red ink, I emerged from the bathroom, minutes later, with it smeared all over my chest and neck. Long story short, I went to dance pink that night.

I was embarrassed and proud all at the same moment as I smiled at my mom and dad, seated across the room. It was Parent Day at dance, and I scrounged every ounce of energy I possessed to hike myself up onto *pointe*.

Uncoordinated, dizzy, weak, and all over the place, I giggled as my mom hugged me after class and told me, "You danced beautifully."

Ah . . . don't you just love moms? Of course, I felt I danced like a hippo giving birth, but Mom convinced me to be happy with trying my best. Many of the other girls' moms called me an "inspiration"—a title I felt I did not deserve, but appreciated nonetheless. I even discovered one girl's mom had done my labs a couple of times. Hmm, it's a small world.

I felt like asking, "What were my counts?"

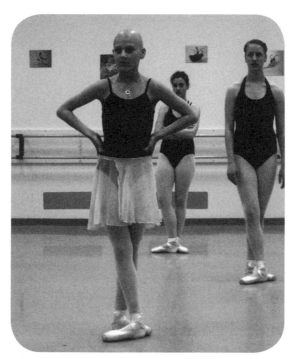

Parent Day at dance 2008 with fellow dancers LaRee and Aniela.

Sprout. That was my new name, referring to the teeny, tiny hairs that now lived upon my head. Every morning, I'd rush to the mirror to see my new growth. Most of the time, I was very cold and bundled up like I was ready for a summit attempt. The baby peach fuzz remained in its own personal "greenhouse" beanie. Maybe that explains its explosive development.

I vividly recall yelling out to Mom, "The main mission of my sprouts is to get darker and find a direction."

Finally, finally the last step was being taken, or at least what I thought was the last step. April twenty-first signaled the start of fourteen days of radiation. This totaled up to be about three weeks, because weekends were treatment free. I probably held my breath as I was lying under the giant stapler-looking machine. Alone in the dim room, I looked around with my eyeballs, careful not to move my head the slightest inch. A fake window that led out to an imaginary garden was painted on the wall to my left, and the roof had those glow in the dark stars you can stick places. Just then, I heard a click.

"Bzzzzzz."

My eyes widened as I saw the plate above me turn from yellow, to orange, to red. I noticed a strange odor—a foul stench that consisted of a mix of burning rubber and chemicals. My chest began to feel hot and tingly, like it had sunburn.

"Whoa, I guess I'm getting radiation," I assumed in my head.

I felt vulnerable. My gown was pulled down to my waist, and I was prone on a pencil-thin table, in the middle of the big room. My trust was exercised to the max. The machine stopped.

"Brrrrrr," the disk above me spun and rotated around a full 180 degrees to my backside. I would be getting radiation from both the front and the back. Afterward, it was kind of creepy, but really fascinating. As I changed out of my gown, I could tell that by the fourteenth time, it was going to be a little old.

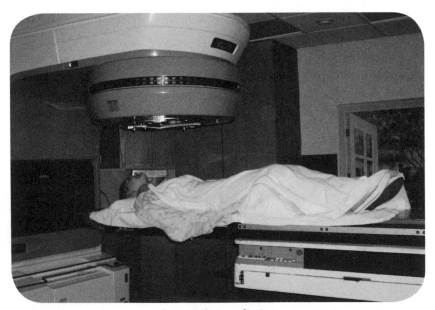

One word . . . radiation.

I decided that I would have to make radiation fun, enjoyable—worth it. So, I got creative. Teddy was dressed in his full Harley Davidson Motorcycle gear, and Little Bear was a cute, cuddly fisherman. They lit up the Cancer Center and, after seeing how much people enjoyed visiting with them, I got an even better idea.

The automatic door slid open, and the three of us strolled into the Cancer Center. I say "three of us," meaning me, my mom, and Antonio, my giant stuffed gorilla. With people's glances, I could pick up his furry, black arm and give a quick wave to those we passed. He sat in the radiation waiting room, occupying his very own chair, occasionally with a magazine sprawled across his wide lap. And then, another idea popped. Dress up time.

Hawaii Antonio wore a pink floral shirt, while bearing leis for Nurse Siobahn and Dr. Weisenburger. Harley Antonio looked rough and tough in his leather jacket, Harley tee, sunglasses, and a bandana wrapped around his head. The reactions only got better as Antonio arrived one day in ballerina attire. A tutu, tights, leotard, and some of my old *pointe* shoes combined to create his hysterical outfit.

The comments were priceless. One woman, outside the hospital, hung out of her van as she drove by, yelling how much she loved him. One day, as he sat in the waiting room, my mom returned from the restroom to find that a crowd had gathered around him. People got to know Antonio. Ed, an extremely kind, loving and comical man from the Cancer Center, became one of Antonio's closest buddies and fans.

He now asks me, "Where's the monkey?" in his slight New York accent when I see him at checkup times.

Popcorn Fridays were Antonio's favorite. He would sit, patiently waiting for me, with a hot, fresh bag of popcorn in his lap. I would place his hand in the bag and stick a piece of popcorn under his upper lip. No one walked by him without at least a grin. Antonio was a man, or, uh, ape of many trades, as the multitude of Antonio Fans could see. He was a superhero one day, complete with underwear and tights, and a doctor the next, clad in full scrubs. Saluting to passersby, one day found Antonio in a patriotic visor and a *Three Stooges* shirt that read, "Curly for President." No one ever knew what he would be wearing tomorrow.

A short time into radiation, my mom and I attended the kickoff event for the Children's Miracle Network. It was a beautiful evening on the patio of State & A, a Santa Barbara restaurant. I sat, after my meal, looking at all the generous people who put their time and effort into this worthy cause. Suddenly, it was him. Dr. Pickert. He began to talk over the speaker and, after saying some very sweet things about me, he introduced me. Not too much longer after this, I found my mom and I having a conversation with him.

"I just always felt like I messed up your sedation," he said, apologetically.

Aw . . . now I felt bad.

"Oh, no, no, no," I corrected him, "stuff happens."

Suddenly, all the times I had poked fun at him were jammed back into my mouth.

"He's *so nice*!" I told Mom as we left the event.

I determined that I could no longer make jokes about him . . . he was way too nice. Darn, he had killed me with kindness. I almost wished he was mean, that way there was an excuse to make fun of him. But he was so cool. Confusion and regret blew off as we walked to our car.

"Crap!" I yelled through my belly laughter. "Why does he have to be *so nice*?"

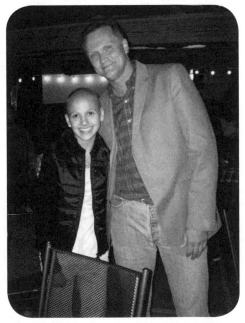

He's so nice! Dr. Pickert and I at the Children's Miracle Network kickoff event.

I'm not sure if the daily drives felt quicker, or longer, as my fourteen days of radiation progressed. Most of the time, I stared out the window looking at the rolling Central California hills and cows chewing their cud. *The Adventures of Huckleberry Finn* played on our car tape player. It was my English schoolwork for those fourteen days. Between my lack of conversation, the narrator's strong dialect, and Mark Twain's creative language, I didn't process much of anything. However, I do remember hearing the phrase "by and by" enough times to make one suicidal. When they weren't saying that, it was repetition of the glorious "n-word" over and over, till my ears burned. I appreciated when the book ended and we were back to listening to the radio.

After daily radiation, I would come home and plop on the couch until dance time. My recital neared, and rehearsals began. Too determined to think straight, I pushed through each exhausting day.

However, going to bed after a long rehearsal, I beamed, exclaiming one night, "I'm so sore!" as I stretched and yawned.

Somehow . . . it felt good.

We approached Butt Hill. And no, that is not a typo. Butt Hill was Mom's and my landmark—our monument. It is a hill that rises out from behind the endless vineyard country and appears to be a . . . well . . . you know. It looked especially special on this day, with horses grazing on its green, flowery "cheeks." But even more special, *this* was my last day of radiation—and treatment.

May 8, 2008, eventually came for me, and as I proudly entered the Cancer Center, I held Antonio in my arms. He wore an apron, a chef's hat, and an oven mitt as he carried a large basket, filled to the brim, with an assortment of freshly baked cookies. For the fourteenth time, I disappeared into the changing room and emerged in my tan, diamond gown that was terribly faded from hundreds of wash and disinfecting sessions.

Mom watched me vanish behind the fish tank, into the dark room with the giant stapler, for the last time. My jaw hung open with surprise as I noticed a makeshift "finish line" and humongous *pointe* shoe balloons. Kym and Sylvia stood bashfully nearby, their eyes clearly displaying the tears that tried to escape. Aw . . . I was going to miss them. It looked like they were going to miss me too, and I pray that I brought a little joy to them in those fourteen days.

A very odd feeling of wanting to be done, but not wanting to be done, confused me as I hopped onto the table. Sitting next to me was a waiting Ballerina Tweety Beanie Baby. Just like my very first blood test, I was once again staring at Tweety—only this time it was all coming to an end, not just all beginning to fall apart. And when that machine wound down for the final time, my soul felt as though it was exploding with joy . . . I had done it. After six long, grueling months, which seemed like years, I had done it. Mom and I exited the Cancer Center, and I hoped that I would never have to be in that horrible, yet hopeful, eerie, yet loving, and frightening, yet comforting place for anything other than a checkup ever again.

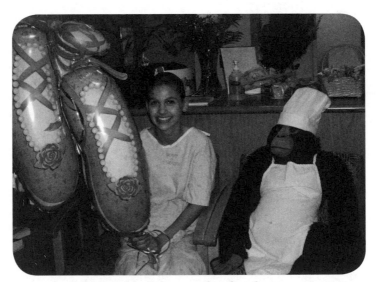

Antonio and I celebrate my last day of treatment.

It was two days after my end of treatment, and a sigh of pure happiness flowed from me as the massive red curtain lifted to a sea of attentive faces. Dead center, and all the way in the back, I felt beautiful in my long peach tutu, *pointe* shoes, and silky, white gloves. This was what I had been waiting for—my recital.

We were the opening dance, and we all knew we had to bring it. Personally, I just prayed that I could get up onto my shoes. My hair was something out of the army . . . somewhere in between a boy cut and bald. So, with my elegant dress, long, sophisticated gloves, and buzz cut, I began to dance the most beautifully I have danced in my life. Of course, I am a million times stronger now, and a much better dancer, but I have never danced with so much feeling, so much passion, and with so much emotion. This was it—I was making my comeback.

I remembered the nights when I would stretch, barely able to bend over to touch my toes. Every muscle hurt me so badly, but I sure didn't care. I recalled the time, shortly after I had gotten my port inserted, that I slipped on my dance shoes and asked my dad to partner, and hold me, as I did a huge, arching *cambre* back on *pointe*. The pain was pretty much unbearable, but I smiled nonetheless. I thought of when I would stand at my kitchen counter in my *pointe* shoes, forcing myself to do thirty-two *relevés* and thirty-two *elevés* in a row, before holding the very last one. I knew I didn't have to do it, but I *wanted* to do it. With so little physical strength, I relied on my mental and spiritual strength to accomplish what I wanted to do.

Suddenly, I heard the music soften . . . it was time for my solo. Running, as gracefully as I could, to center stage, I began to dance as I felt the music more and more. I was the music, and the music was me. We have always been close to each other. Even at the tender age of one, my chin would quiver, and tears would flow down my chipmunk cheeks, as my mom sang hymns to me. When my dad would play a song on the piano, I would lie on the couch nearby, silently crying into a pillow. Church was the worst. Every song touched me to the point of tears. Music has always been *so* beautiful to me. I not only *hear* it, I also *feel* it deep down in my soul. To me, there is an emotion behind each and every note and tone—a purpose.

So, during those thirty seconds of pure heaven, I felt so happy, so incredible, and so proud. I didn't have to say a word; my dancing said everything. With a big leap, my short solo came to an end, but what happened at that moment was unreal. Applause broke out, and I looked and saw all of my friends, my family, and people I barely knew, on their feet—for me. They all love me so much, and words cannot say how much that moment meant to me. To look out and see the faces of all the people who got me through my battle was just too good to be true. They smiled and cheered for me . . . all because they cared about me. The love that surrounded me was too big to fit in the whole auditorium.

Life stood still at that second, and I felt like God was telling me, "*Well done, Melinda. Now go and dance.*"

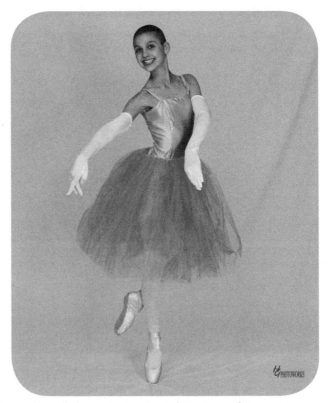

Hancock Youth Dance Spring Recital 2008, two days post-treatment.
Photo by Heidi Gruetzemacher, Photoworks Frame Gallery.

It was party time. Having had a long day, I was ready to celebrate. After my recital, my family hosted an End of Treatment and Thank You BBQ, with seventy-six of our friends and family, right after my recital ended. To be able to physically hug all of those who supported me through everything was the best part. People swam in our pool, laughed, played cards around the tables, and ate the delicious food that Ric, our longtime neighbor, busily cooked. Arriving with his giant, pit BBQ, towing behind his big, diesel truck, he would take no money, but wanted to do it out of the kindness of his own heart.

The love at that party was unbelievable, and people who had never even met clicked instantly because of their similar purpose for being there—they cared about me. Even Dr. Dan and his family drove all the way from his Santa Barbara home. Our dog, Larry, was chased and petted the whole time by his small children, Jake and Aliyah, who absolutely adored him. I gave Dr. Dan a gift, hand drawn, from whom else, but me. It was a drawing of the clinic, and it included Nanci, Zippy, Nurse Pam, Robyn, and, of course . . . Dr. Dan.

To my surprise, a stack of gifts waited on our living room table. I was overwhelmed—didn't know what to say. Plopping on the couch as the party wound down, exhaustion yet pure joy mixed to form my unique expression. At that moment, I didn't know how life could get any better.

"Many other women have kicked higher, balanced longer, or turned faster. These are poor substitutes for passion." —**Agnes de Mille**

SEVENTEEN

THERE WAS A PROBLEM . . . a big problem. After reaching the climax, I had, once again, sunk down into the daily battle with feeling ill.

Many, including myself, think, "Poof! I'm done!"

"Whooptidoo! On with life!"

Ohhhh . . . no. I don't think so. I still felt sick.

"What kind of crud is this?" I thought.

The phrase, "*done* with treatment," has an invisible, "and now the long recovery process begins," attached to the end of it that I slowly began to realize. They shouldn't use the words, "done," "end," or "finished" . . . because it's the beginning of a whole separate maze of obstacles. I found myself sitting around doing absolutely *nothing*, still feeling exactly the same I had felt all along. Only this time, though, it was more frustrating because it seemed like there was no goal, no end to it all.

At least during treatment, I had something to strive for, to reach for—the end of treatment. Now I was there, and I sat bitterly on the couch, realizing just how much it stunk. At least during treatment, I felt like I was taking the necessary steps to make a full recovery, but now, I was lost—completely lost. A whole life sprawled out in front of me, and I had no freakin' idea what to do with it. I strongly considered just lying on the couch in front of the TV until some magical, nonexistent day came when I was myself again. My mind was just . . . blah. Treatment had been pretty brutal, I'm not gonna lie, but I was starting to think that recovery was even worse.

Life only got more difficult as I began to experience late effects from treatment. Eating became a huge struggle, and my previous love of food started to turn into a hateful relationship. My stomach was tiny, and I would feel extremely, and uncomfortably, full after little food. Everything hurt, and I was scared and anxious before eating for fear of how it would make me feel.

Lying on our living room floor, I remember holding my belly while it tortured me. I didn't think it was fair that I had to go through more pain . . . I didn't think I should have to suffer anymore. Feeling like my body was still my enemy . . . I fought, beginning to hate it more and more, until I considered it evil. Really, all that it wanted me to do was rest it, nourish it, and nurture it, but I was still in battle mode. My switch was broken—busted—and I had no concept or intention of giving in to my body. After having it put me through hell, I felt it was *my* turn.

The portal for my spirit had been cherished, taken care of, and loved at one time, but now, it was just a thing to me. I believe I was in search of something to blame for all of my suffering and felt that since it was my body that hurt so badly and felt so sick, then *it* must be what was slowly sucking my joy away. Honestly, I didn't even really care about what happened to my body anymore, or what it went through. Fighting each brutal moment, the anger and frustration stacked up inside of me. The very last thing I thought to give my body was food. It wanted food, and what it wanted, I was not about to let it have—it would only hurt me in return.

Seeing in the rearview mirror that my eyelashes were finally growing back, I admired the small stubbles protruding from my eyelids. After the thirty-minute car ride, we reached our destination and my excitement skyrocketed as we pulled into a little parking lot at the end of a cul-de-sac. The huge sign on the side of the building read:

"More than Ever, now is the time to Dance."

Yep, this was my kind of place, the Academy of Dance. With spontaneous energy created by my bubbly anxiousness, Mom and I entered and approached the instructor. Her name is Michelle, and she introduced herself with one of the sweetest, and most sincere, smiles I have ever witnessed. I had read about her in the studio's brochure that I had jammed in Mom's hands and asked her to look over. My sad eyes must have convinced Mom that I still needed dance during my summer break.

Anyway, Michelle had danced with the Joffrey Ballet . . . that was *big*, no, *huge*. Not only is she an incredible dancer, but a person with a heart of gold, as my mom and I both became aware of quite quickly. Looking back, I now feel silly having been so borderline starstruck.

I guess I just dreamed so passionately about transforming into an even better dancer than before. Literally, I would lie in my own puddle of misery, the tears flowing faster with each painful sob, and picture myself dancing. Strong, healthy, and happy, I would gently glide across the clouds in my own head. I saw a Melinda who was not chained down and held back by her own body . . . she was free to dance to her heart's content.

So, as I stood looking up at Michelle, that's what I did, *look up* to her. She was everything I wanted, prayed, fought, and worked to be. Health, strength, and joyfulness—that's all I wanted, and it all stood before me, combined to form one magnificent person. Immediately, I felt like a little kid looking up to her hero.

"I want to be just like you," I thought to myself.

Feeling somewhat intimidated and weak in her presence, it also gave me more determination to work even harder. Class began, and I found myself trying not to look like, well, a girl fresh out of cancer treatments. Mom had told Michelle about my unique situation, but, as always, I did not want to use my illness as an excuse for doing something halfway. Over my dead body was I going to give myself permission to *not* give it my best, but when my fragile body just could not quite do something, I forced myself to let it slide, despite my frustration.

For the most part, I was very excited, but at the same time, I couldn't help but wonder how the other girls would treat me. I hoped that they wouldn't judge me by my dancing before they knew who I really was. Smiling at my mom, watching in the corner, I molded my attitude into what was favorable at the time.

It was my "Here I am. This is the best I can do, and I'm just happy to be dancing" attitude.

Fortunately, I discovered the girls were the sweetest people on Earth, creating a feeling of family and support within the small studio.

And as I exited the studio, hot and tired, yet beaming, I told Mom, "The girls all look so familiar . . . like I've seen them before. I mean, they look so familiar!"

My mom turned to me, grinning. "They do to me too."

Driving away in a state of puzzlement, I wondered how, and why, it all felt so right there. A perfect fit—an identical match . . . I was going to like it there.

Fatigue affected me *everywhere*. With my body incessantly feeling like a glop of mud, I began to notice that my brain, too, was turning to mush. School became a nightmare. I sat on the floor, with my book open, my eyes squinting in the morning light.

"All cells have outer coverings," I read.

Seeing the words, and reading the words, I suddenly realized I had absolutely no idea what they meant.

"Focus, Melinda! Focus," I thought to myself before concentrating even harder.

"All cells have outer coverings."

What did that mean?! It was just words—no meaning, no connection—*nothing*. Anger stewed inside of me. *Why* couldn't I think? What was going on? I had been able to just *read* before, and now, suddenly, I felt like a preschooler. Taking a deep breath, I resorted to a somewhat drastic technique.

"All," I read.

Okay, I got it. That meant every one of them.

"Cells," I continued.

Alright, those were the little dudes that we're made of. Picturing a small, round cell, I fought to retain the image.

"All cells," okay, okay, "all cells."

Let's see, "have," that means that they've got something.

Okay, okay.

"All cells have," I reread.

I thought I was finally getting it.

"Outer coverings."

Hmm. Picturing my cell again, I imagined a . . . something around it, though I couldn't quite see it fully.

"Oh, a covering! A covering!"

It suddenly clicked.

"All cells have outer coverings!" I read, proudly.

I then held the image of a pea-shaped sphere in my mind, with a thin shell surrounding it. After securing it in my memory bank, I felt it was safe to move on.

"It is called the cell membrane and is composed of a lipid bi-layer and protein channels."

Crud. Here we go again.

With the twenty-ninth of May came a giant fourteen. Yep, I was fourteen years old, and didn't quite feel my age. To be honest, I was extremely confused, feeling like a two-year-old one day and a senior citizen the next. Wishing that, for at least my birthday, I could be free from feeling ill, I at last came to terms of acceptance that I would feel cruddy on my birthday.

However, I have good memories of the events of the day. Mom and I had some quality time together at the beach and, afterward, did a little shopping. We met up with the family later to see *Indiana Jones* before going back to our place for a few presents. I was grateful I had made it to fourteen, but sad I barely got a chance to be thirteen.

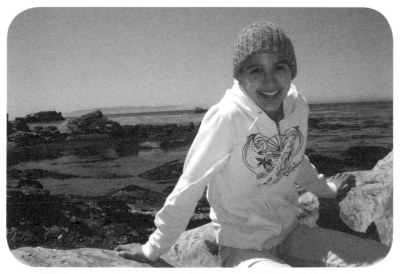

Celebrating my fourteenth birthday at the Shell Beach tidepools.

☞

Walking onto the set, a man pointed to the camera I would speak to. Another man who looked like he had authority, sat behind the film crew and counted down the seconds before going live. I was being interviewed for the Children's Miracle Network Telethon; in fact, my whole family was. The hospital was in full bloom, with banners, signs, and even a giant, more than life size poster of me in the cafeteria.

Glenn, the hospital photographer, and I had a photo shoot one day before the telethon. It was slightly overwhelming for my exhausted body and mind to be there, but I was no less thrilled to be giving back to the place that had, well, saved me. I felt it was my duty, my calling, and it felt incredible to finally use all that I'd gone through for good. Those who came after me would have state-of-the-art . . . everything to treat them, if I had anything to say about it.

Expressing my excitement for being at the event, I smiled back at a local newsman who interviewed me. I went on to tell the story of a cleaning man who sang to me during my fourth round. Describing his golden voice, which sang a beautiful Spanish song, I was spiritually brought back to that very day. It was people like him, I said, that make Cottage Hospital special.

Mom, Dad, Nicholas, and Dean added a few words, and within a snap of a finger, it was over. I hoped that someone had seen my story and interview and wanted to call in to make a donation. Right as the thought drifted out of my mind, I heard a phone ring, and a volunteer answered with a smile. That was it. It was worth it to me at that moment. My cancer had a meaning—a purpose. It was doing what I thought it was not capable of doing—giving.

☞

Thousands of memories, feelings, hopes, and dreams all formed the three scrolls of paper that were clutched in my hand. Warmth from the blazing fire softly skimmed my face, diminishing the frigid night air. Moms, dads, brothers, and sisters sat crowded around with their very own cancer kid, the dancing flames lighting up their solemn faces. June had finally snuck onto my calendar, and my mom and I were at the American Cancer Society's Camp Reach for the Stars. We stood close together, manufacturing both love and warmth on the cool, coastal night. Nobody talked, except for a few who wished to share what they had written for the fire ceremony. The kids' hopes, dreams, and wishes were all written on small scrolls before throwing them into the fire to "release them up to the stars."

I had written that I wished for nothing but love and peace in the world, health and happiness for me and my family, and, of course, to be able to dance forever and ever and ever. There was a brief moment before the scroll disintegrated completely in the hot flames. You could also create a scroll in memory of someone, and tears filled my glassy eyes as I clutched my second paper roll.

"G-pop. This is for you, buddy. I love you," I thought, peering up at the glowing stars on the clear, crisp night.

"Look. I made it, G-pop. I made it, buddy. I sure wish you were here to celebrate with me, but I have no doubt you're perched on one of those stars, smiling down right now. I love you, G-pop."

His scroll dropped into the fire, and his memory floated straight to where he sat. Looking down at the last remaining paper, my tears began to flow even faster—even harder.

My Great-Aunt Marion passed away May twenty-seventh . . . two days prior to my birthday. Cancer. Cancer had taken her away from us. During my battle, I had been the closest to her that I had ever been before because of our cancer kinship. She left me loving messages on my CarePage and sent me cards. I was amazed that someone in such poor health could be so selfless, but likewise, I did the same.

Closing my eyes for a moment, I took the time to remember when I had sent a gift to her. She was not doing well at all, and I felt it a duty as a, what I began to call "chemo buddy," that I should be there for her. Selecting and purchasing the prettiest box I could find at the post office, I filled it to the brim with nearly everything to make a person feel good. A hand-knitted bag was filled with goodies to brighten her day. The card I included told her how much I loved her and that if my "chemo buddy" needed anything, I was there for her. I told her to stay strong, and together, we would beat it. I made it on the computer, complete with a backdrop of clouds and angels.

My favorite quote, "*We are all angels with one wing, we can only fly by embracing one another,*" was on the front cover, under a big red heart.

Her son, Jason, later told me that my card remained right by her bedside until her death. When she died, I felt as though a part of my strength went missing, like one of my pillars had been knocked down. A million memories of her raced through my mind as her scroll slid into the fire and was suddenly gone—lost forever. This was exactly how it was with G-pop and Aunt Marion—they were forever gone out of our lives, yet the feelings, the memories, and remembrances would always be there to comfort me.

My tears welled up as others grieved their own losses, and small, sick children sent their dreams soaring to the heavens. In that fire burned a million stories, and an invisible pile of love, sadness, hope, and strength stood beneath the golden flames.

⌒

I wasn't eating. Literally, I was *not eating*. At the camp, I had eaten nothing other than fruit. I didn't want to, nor did I let myself, eat anything else. My stomach bothered me nonstop, and as I stepped on the clinic's scale on June ninth, I weighed eighty-seven pounds, ten less than when I started. Dr. Dan was not extremely concerned and explained that with each step of recovery, I would gain back healthy weight.

"Not if I have anything to say about it," I thought.

Control over many things, especially my body, was beginning to create an obsessive fear with losing control. A glimpse of what was really important hit me when Dr. Dan reported that my chest X-ray and PET/CT were all clear. I was happy, yet for some odd reason, I felt like I was forcing myself to be happy. Of course, it was what I wanted, and I prayed that nothing would return, but a weird sort of anger, and feeling I cannot possibly describe, was within me.

This is when things began to steadily shred apart—my life became a mudslide, and I clawed my way to the surface, which only sucked me down deeper and deeper. Depression I was not fully aware of left me in a ball on the floor, where I cried until my eyes stung and my head throbbed. Feeling like my life, and all that made me happy, was slowly being wrenched away from me, I started to question why I had fought . . . and if it was even worth it.

⌒

With my digestive problems continuing and worsening, Dr. Dan sent me down the hall for an appointment with Dr. Kelts, the pediatric gastroenterologist. As I described my symptoms, he looked confidently at me from behind his round glasses. Yep, he had seen it a million times. Constipation. He explained that, with all of the medications I had been taking, I had become "clogged up." It made me sick, picturing hundreds of pills forming a mini-dam in my intestines. Ewww.

So, Dr. Kelts gave me the usual "Drink more water," and he also instructed me to eat "poopy foods," aka old people, fiber food.

Praying that we had located my problem, I somehow knew that it was not what was causing me so much pain. However, feeling so depressed, I couldn't think correctly. I just waited for some miracle.

☞

I could see the earthy, green Washington trees out of the studio's small window. That's right, my mom and I were in Washington State. A friend's daughter was getting married, and I was away for, really, the very first trip since getting sick. Our friend Johanna has another daughter, Madisen, who is passionate about dance, almost as much as me. And so, when the idea came up about me taking a class at her studio, I ran to the bathroom and changed into my leotard and tights quicker than a cheetah.

Approaching the woodsy studio, I was brimming with excitement. The teacher, I had been told, was a dancer with the Pacific Northwest Ballet, the same company that my beloved Patricia Barker had danced with. Wow, I got to not only *dance* on my vacation but also have a professional as my instructor. I was determined to hang tight. Good thing, too, because she was tough, and *mean*. Really *mean*. However, I'm pretty good when it comes to people like that, so I took it with a grain of salt. After forty minutes or so doing *barre*, we began doing *centre* work.

I was thrilled when I landed one double *pirouette* after another, as the other girls who frequented the studio wore inquisitive expressions.

"Where did *she* come from?"

However, I tired quickly.

After Miss Sunshine taught the jump combo, I hit a nice fifth position and prepared to work hard. With beat after beat, I pushed to finish the combination. Meanwhile, Miss Congeniality yelled at us from the corner, making us do right, left, right *again*, and, once again, left. Upon our completion, she immediately stated her disappointment and commanded us to do it again. Ugh. I was getting tired—*really* tired. My focus and drive that day must have been incredible, though, because there I went again, redoing the entire thing, with the hope of somehow pleasing her.

Proudly stretching out after the brutal combo, my heart fell to the floor as I heard these words: "Do it again!"

A class-wide groan erupted, except from me, who only silently stepped forward to, once again, give it a shot. I have to admit, I was a little worried, I mean—I was so freakin' exhausted—I was *beyond* fatigued. The music started, and my body just went.

"I can do it, I can do it," I thought, with each jolting bounce and every thigh-burning beat.

Suddenly, I noticed everything . . . I began to think way too much.

"Wait," I thought, "I'm straight out of cancer treatment . . . how can my body do all this? I'm nuts! She's gonna kill me!"

Air pounded in and out of my lungs, but it was still not enough. I felt like I couldn't breathe, no, wait, I really *couldn't breathe*. Stopping right in the middle of it all, I rushed toward the door, where my mom sat outside in the small room. Bursting through, I painfully wheezed as I held my chest. Poor Mom nearly had a heart attack as she watched me collapse into a chair with a terrified expression on my pale face. For a moment, I thought I had really stopped breathing. The feeling of wanting and needing to breathe, but being unable to do so, is eerie and frightening beyond words. Focusing on taking nice, deep breaths, I began to recover. I felt so bad for my mom, who only stood next to me, unaware of what had happened. When she asked if she should call an ambulance, I instantly pictured one racing through the woods to save me.

"No, no, no, I'm fine," I reassured her through my gasps.

"Are you sure?!" she questioned, the horror and worry shining on her face.

"Yeah, I just need to sit here for a sec," I replied, trying to be the calmest I could for fear of freaking her out even further.

We sat in silence for a few minutes, with nothing but the sound of my frantic pants and the music penetrating the door. Oh my gosh . . . they were doing it *again*, and apparently, they didn't miss me much.

I started to calm down, and air flowed with more and more ease, yet I still created a strange respiratory sound. Looking out the window near me, I acknowledged the stunning trees and also noticed something else.

"Look!" I yelled excitedly to Mom, "a bunny!"

She lowered her head and, after rubbing her tired face, displayed her disbelief with a slow shake of her head.

It was a "What am I gonna do with you?" moment.

When Mom determined it was safe, we departed—leaving the bunny and Adolf Hitler of the Ballet World behind.

"Dance first. Think later. It's the natural order." —Samuel Beckett

EIGHTEEN

RETURNING HOME from our trip, things got bad—extremely bad. My depression haunted me every second of every day. I didn't want to do anything anymore. I didn't get joy out of anything, and I began to think that life was too painful—too hard. At some point during each and every day, an emotional breakdown occurred, and I would end up on the floor, while my brothers and Dad distanced themselves from me. I guess it was way too much for them to see me like that. Misery. Hell. Evil. That is how I describe this point in my journey. I felt as though I didn't even really exist, but just constantly lived in a bubble of each and every emotion I possessed. Mom and I both would say that we believed we would not fall apart until after treatment . . . we were right.

Suddenly, I experienced an overwhelming amount of feelings surfacing within me. Anger about things that did not even faze me at the time transformed me into a person neither my family nor I recognized. There was so much pain, so much suffering, within me I could not stand it any longer.

Why? Why did I have to be so scarred, so haunted, so disturbed by all that I had gone through?

Only pushing through it at the time, I did not expect the fear, anger, and desperation to arise months and months later. Now, I *felt* my pain; I *felt* my frustration. It was as if God had simply spared me the suffering during treatment so that I would be able to fight. The severity of all I had gone through left my mind in another world, one where all is dark, and nothing can pull you out except God Himself.

Standing, facing our living room wall, I would lean my head against it, and I would just *stand* there. For literally over half an hour, I would enter some strange planet of anger and evil and darkness. What was happening to me? I felt that when I was smiling and happy, I was forcing it upon myself—putting on an act. But at home, my mask came off, and my deep, deep emotional, physical, and spiritual pain isolated me from the entire world. People would tell me I "looked great," but I was frustrated with the fact that I had no words to tell them how much I was suffering inside. A sick emptiness weighed me down wherever I went—a hole that cancer slowly drilled deeper and wider in my heart, with each piece of my life it took away.

This couldn't be happening. How did this happen? What do I do? The endless questions that filled my mind only frustrated me more. My mom was the only one who remained very close to me during this time. I talked to her sometimes, but at other times, I just couldn't find words to express my deep thoughts. My thoughts would scare even me. The abyss to which my mind's thoughts dove only sank me deeper into depression.

Another occurrence that bothered me was when others would ask how I was doing. Of course, I was appreciative of their concern, but I found myself struggling for an answer. I always said "good," but realized one day that I was flat-out lying. Not wanting to burden people with my own problems, I also, honestly, wouldn't know where to start to answer their question. I'd have them there for a good week.

"Mom," I asked one day, as I expressed my concern in this area "how do I tell people, 'Well, today I was baking a quiche, got frustrated, threw something across the room, cursed, and then cried'?"

You can see my dilemma.

Food was a delicate subject. I felt "fat," aka, sick, weak, worthless, and helpless, all rolled into one three-letter-word. Basically, it meant I was not happy with who I was. I wanted to have "me" back. Bitterness enclosed my every thought, and I knew inside I would not be happy until my life was back in my own hands. What I really needed to do was ride out the tidal wave, be patient, and make the best out of what was thrown at me, but I became determined to fix everything myself.

This has always been both my strength and my weakness—determination. The drive I possess can help me accomplish almost anything, yet, I am extremely hard on myself when those goals are not quite reached, even by my best effort. I never give myself a break.

☙

During this time, it was by no means an obsession with being perfect but, rather, a mix between impatience and a search for self-worth—reassurance that I should still be among the living. Determination to feel good about me began to morph into an eating disorder, and my physical digestive problems did not assist whatsoever in the matter. I just wanted to *feel good* . . . inside and out. Health and happiness—that's all I really wanted.

As I would look into the mirror at my rapidly shrinking body, something would make me feel good. That sensation of absolutely *nothing* in my stomach gave me an almost high and a sick sort of happiness. But that happiness quickly turned inside-out and only added to the hole in my spirit. I had no concept of portion sizes . . . nothing. At best, a peach was breakfast. Maybe, if I exercised, I would get an apple and dry cereal for lunch. I was my own Drill Sergeant, my own enemy. Feeling trapped and victimized, I also, strangely, felt powerful and in control. Only now do I realize that I was not only killing my body, but my spirit as well. Now, knowing that all I really wanted at the end of the day was to curl up in front of the TV with a full belly and my family, I feel stupid—ashamed.

I gave myself no relief—allowed myself no joy—except for those few moments where "I deserved it."

Those moments only came after strenuous exercise, or a day of fasting. Then, my body's bloody screams would result in me devouring a whole box of crackers or cereal before I collapsed on the floor, sobbing in hysterics. For so long, I did not forgive myself. Hating my life, I did not realize *I* was the one who was making it so miserable. The negative energy that poisoned my body was being used to do something I never should have done. But when I saw those bones sticking out further and further . . . the sick pleasure would return to me . . . and keep me along the path to self-destruction.

☙

I was pissed. I would have to miss dance. Plopped on our couch, I chugged down another glass of "Go-lightly." It was the fifth, no, the sixth . . . seventh? I wasn't sure. I had lost count. With my stomach and intestinal problems continuing to worsen, Dr. Kelts called in the heavy duty stuff. Go-lightly is used before people get a colonoscopy, to, well, you know. I groaned at the site of the gallon jug in our fridge that was, still, well over half full. Instructed to drink the whole thing as fast as I could, I was nearly about to barf a quarter of the way through. My tiny stomach stretched up to the moon as I reclined on the couch, taking one nauseating sip after another.

Nurse Pam had told me it was going to be a movie day.

"Lay there, pause, run to the bathroom, and repeat."

I don't think I ate anything the entire day because of my bloated stomach, which made me look pregnant. Ugh, I felt obese . . . disgusting. The salty tasting liquid gurgled inside of me. Ugh. And then, I began to become one with the potty. I felt *terrible*, but for some odd reason, my sick mind somewhat enjoyed it. Everything was gone, out, and that's the way I wanted it. I can't believe I am writing this now, but it felt kind of good to me. I knew then that it shouldn't, and it scared me that it did.

That night, I began to feel very weird. I remained awake later than usual because of the toilet-related matters. As I sat in front of the TV, I noticed my head began to have an eerie, spinning sensation. My vision seemed funny, and my body felt weak and tingly. Sighing, I made my way to the kitchen. I thought that I must need food. Munching on crackers, I noticed that I was not feeling better, but almost worse. I became slightly frightened . . . I had never felt this way before. What was it?

My anxiety built, and I hurried to the kitchen again, returning seconds later with a bowl of cheese. Eating like I had not seen food in a year, I devoured the entire thing. Ugh. I felt like a pig. Suddenly, I realized it had not helped . . . I felt even sicker. Okay, now I was scared.

Chugging a glass of milk, I concluded it tasted horrible and rued my decision. Oh, I drank it with my prednisone back in the day. Whoa, nothing was working. I told Mom, and she stood nearby as I brushed my teeth, preparing for bed.

Maybe I just needed a good night's sleep. Yeah, I bet that would fix things. But my tension grew, and I finally allowed myself to truly assess how I was feeling—unbelievably horrific.

"I *really* don't feel well," I admitted to Mom, trying to stay calm.

Dropping my toothbrush with a thud, I asked Mom to help me to bed.

"I'm *freezing*," I told her as she raced to retrieve blankets.

"I've never felt like this before," I whispered, my face turning pale.

"Should we go to the emergency room?" Mom asked, with the same expression I had witnessed in Washington.

"I don't know, I don't know. I'm kinda scared," I confessed.

I began to experience the worst chills of my life, and I started to involuntarily shake. My wide eyes focused on the yellow ceiling. I fought to remain conscious.

"I'm really scared," I announced, with a mummified face.

My mom held my hand as I fought each brutal moment.

"I want to go to the ER, Mom. I'm scared. I'm scared."

It was true. Never in my life had I been so helplessly terrified. A feeling of darkness swept over me. I felt myself fading, the vision of my mom becoming less clear with each second. I felt death, and no words can be used to describe the emotions I experienced.

"No! No!" I screamed inside my head.

"&*@$#, no! I'm not gonna die! I'm not gonna *%$@# die!"

Mom let go of my hand.

"No, I need you," I thought.

She would have to run to the window and call out to the spa for my dad's help. Nicholas was already in bed, and Dean was out with Dad. Concentrating so hard to relax and take nice, deep breaths, I heard my mom's cries for help. Confusion mounted as Dean and my dad entered to find me barely hanging on. I couldn't talk or move. I feared it would require too much energy . . . and that would be it. My unintentional shaking mixed with a deathly bone chill, despite the mountain of blankets covering me.

Just then, I faintly saw Dean, who took my hand with a firm hold. Squeezing back, I found it helped me to remain awake. My worst fear, at that moment, was slipping away from him, sliding into an unconscious state. At so many moments, I braced in fear, praying to God to help me stay here. I imagine that is what people feel like when they die . . . slipping, fading, slowing traveling to an unknown darkness as the world dissolves around them.

I was so focused. Staring into my brother's eyes, I fought hard to be there with him. His hand's warm grasp was the only thing that comforted me. His hand was worth more than all the money in the world to me at that moment, and I periodically squeezed it when I felt myself fading. Somehow, it always brought me back.

My dad, shocked and stumbling around aimlessly, got some orders from Dean.

"Dad!" he told him. "Get the blankets."

With who knows how much red wine running through his bloodstream, Dad was still wandering.

"Dad," Dean spoke even louder. "Get the blankets!"

Still, nothing sunk in.

"Dad," Dean yelled this time. "Get the f@#%* blankets!"

Dad finally got the picture.

Mom and dad quickly changed their clothes, and I suddenly felt myself lifted off of the bed as Dean carried me to the car. Cradled in his arms . . . I felt so thankful for him, but was left unable to share my feelings.

The car ride was a battle in itself. The same roads we had traveled hundreds of times suddenly looked different, darker, and even more eerie. And when we arrived at Marion Hospital's ER, I could not believe where I was and what was happening. Everything was a blur as my dad pushed me in a wheelchair through the sliding doors, with at least ten blankets piled on top of me. I still shook. Mom was parking the car; she had driven on account of Dad having gotten pretty toasty with his wine out in the spa that night.

I realized the severity of his toastiness when he turned to me and inquired, "When's your birthday?"

Wow, you have got to be kidding me.

"5/29/94," I recited, after finding the strength to reply.

"Oh, and what's your Social Security number?"

This was a joke—a complete disaster. Yeah, leave it to my tipsy dad to sign me in.

"I don't know!" I replied, the frustration quite apparent in my voice.

Here I was . . . filling in the gaps the alcohol had made in my dad's brain. I was not sure whether to laugh or cry.

When Mom arrived, she told them I was a cancer patient, and I got in almost immediately. The ER tripped me out as I was rolled in and approached an empty room. The equipment looked serious . . . I prayed they wouldn't have to use it. After a short examination by the doctor, and a brief explanation from my parents, an IV dug into my arm as I winced in pain. The world's biggest bag of fluids began to drain into me. I was severely dehydrated—to the point of shock from lack of fluids.

The Go-lightly had sucked everything out of me, almost the life out of me. I was sent back home. Arriving around midnight, I found myself exhausted. A giant glass of water sat an arm's reach away, and I woke frequently and suddenly in the night to take a gulp. Promising myself to drink more water, I prayed I would never have to go through what I went through ever again. I despised Go-lightly, and when Dr. Dan asked me about it at my next visit, my response was swift.

"Go-lightly! Pfff! More like Go-heavily!"

I now realize that on that night, July seventh, my life could very well have been taken away from me.

A feeling of pride came over me as I flowed among the slow-moving crowd of purple T-shirts. On the back of each one was written "Survivor," and I was one of them. Each person in the sea of hope that walked around the school's track held their own story of downfall, battle, and victory. As I completed the Relay for Life's Survivor Lap, I found my heart pouring out gratitude to God, to Dr. Dan, to anyone and anything on Earth. Seeing the other people walking beside me, I could tell they all felt the same exact way. We had all been there, and our immediate kinship created a powerful, yet silent, feeling among us. It was also amazing to witness those generous, selfless people who weren't survivors but who gave their time because of a family member's or friend's life touched by cancer, or just a concern for the cause. Two of those caring people were my Gramma and Poppy. Honestly, I wished I could hug each and every one of them . . . those who donated their money, or their efforts, tucked themselves into the pockets of my heart. They were my inspirations, my heroes.

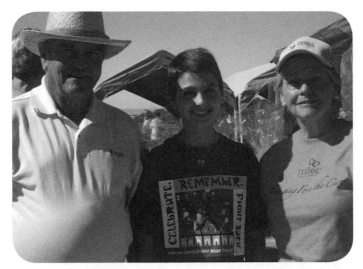

Gramma, Poppy, and I walk for the cure at the Arroyo Grande Relay for Life 2008.

One of these people was a man named Zac, who works for Jamba Juice. A booth was set up, and he and a woman named Jamie were selling smoothies, with all of the proceeds going straight to the American Cancer Society. My mom and I walked around the track, and suddenly, a giant, yellow . . . something came up behind us. It was a banana—a man in a banana suit with a tray of smoothies in his arms. Zac smiled and waved to us, dancing to the music that blared over the PA system.

"Hey! Banana Man," I yelled, as I too began to get jiggy.

He noticed my Survivor shirt, and we got to talking. His enthusiasm was contagious.

"Hey," he called back to me as our conversation ended, "come by the booth later, and I'll get you a smoothie on me!"

Wow, what a cool guy, I thought. He was out there, giving up his day, selling his smoothies, and wearing a *banana suit*. But what really got me was his joy, his spark, and his sincere smile. He danced, made people laugh, and created a fun and loving atmosphere around him—all things he really didn't have to do.

Mom took a picture of me, Zac, and Jamie. We blew it up, framed it, and later gave it to them with cards and home baked banana bread, of course! So now, every time I walk into Jamba Juice in Arroyo Grande, I look up at our picture on the wall and say hi to my friends, Jamie and Banana Man.

That night was special. Holding my mom's hand, I slowly crept along the edge of the track while silence engulfed the entire event. It was becoming darker with each second, the sun disappearing below the horizon. With the darkness came the iridescent glow of the hundreds of luminary bags that lined the path. My grasp still tight, we read the bags one by one.

"In memory. In memory. In memory."

With each one, my spirit sank lower and lower.

"Papa, we love you, and we miss you."

The messages broke my heart, piece by piece. We came to the bag I had decorated "In Memory of" Aunt Marion, and we stopped in front of it—tears beginning to form in my eyes. The picture of her glowed from the inside out, with the candle's soft, flickering light. It looked beautiful . . . she looked beautiful.

Next, we came to my Great-Aunt Phyllis's bag, another one I had decorated. This one, thankfully, was "In Honor of." She was my other chemo buddy, and I had sent her a gift box too. Standing by her twinkling bag, I felt so happy for her . . . she did it. We did it—together.

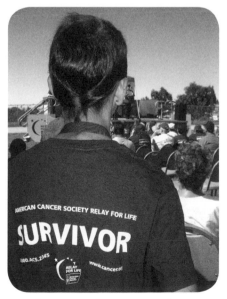

A moment of so many emotions.

Lastly, we approached one more bag, my bag. Amid a sea of "In Memory of" bags stood mine, a single survivor in a line of lost lives. Guilt, I felt guilt. Why had I made it? Why hadn't they? Overwhelming gratitude, yet sadness, created a strange concoction of emotions within me. I didn't think it was fair for them. They deserved life, and I suddenly didn't care if God switched me out with one of them. But I didn't want to die, nor did I want *them* to die. It was all so confusing.

Why was I here? Had I fought harder? Or did God just keep me here for some reason? And, if so, what is that reason?

"At times our own light goes out and is rekindled by a spark from another person. Each of us has cause to think with deep gratitude of those who have lighted the flame within us."
—Albert Schweitzer

NINETEEN

IT WAS NOW AUGUST, and I finally finished Lance Armstrong's book, *It's Not about the Bike*. Okay, he was, officially, the coolest person on the globe, and my *total* hero and inspiration. I learned that Lance and I have a lot in common, more than you would think. We have the same drive, the same internal push that can sometimes result in self-harming ways. Our determination surpasses our physical SOS signals, and we both have an unbelievable passion for our "sports"—cycling and dancing. Plus, we both beat cancer and made our comebacks—defying the odds. Okay, well, I was still making my comeback, but that's beside the point. Thinking about how cool it would be to meet him one day made me smile and giggle.

"Who knows?" I thought.

The impossible could happen . . . I knew that by then.

As I transitioned onto stage, in my bright blue unitard and black skirt, I felt weak, but happy. I was able to perform in a dance for the Academy of Dance's annual school show in August. Trying to execute every movement, I noticed that my stomach felt hollow and empty—perfect. I had purposely not eaten anything so that I would feel . . . not well, but better than if I ate.

Sitting in the back of the dressing room after I had finished, I watched the other girls rushing everywhere, costumes flying left and right. It looked fun. I wanted to be in a ton of dances like them, barely concluding one before sprinting backstage to begin another. Ah, yeah . . . that was the life. Alone in the quiet dressing room, I imagined myself with so many costumes, I could barely keep them all straight. Ha, and there I sat in what I had come in, what I danced in, and what I would leave in.

I pictured myself hot and sweaty, with the bright dressing room lights feeling like a bunch of tiny suns, only making me hotter. In reality, I was not only bone dry, I hadn't even come close to breaking a sweat—I was cold. The chills ran through me as I sat and waited, feeling rather stupid. My breathing felt as shallow as a puddle, and as some of the girls returned to the room, I looked at them with a weird sort of envy. They appeared so healthy, so strong . . . which made me seem even sicker, even weaker.

A ball on the floor or my leaning-head-against-the-wall pose—those had become my two life positions. After every single meal, the floor was my spot. Curled up the tightest I possibly could, I would sob and sob for what seemed like an eternity. Holding my stomach, I strongly desired to rip it out . . . it would hurt less. At times, I would just scream. I honestly didn't know what else to do. I felt disturbed, sad, and so angry inside, and the things that tormented me physically tortured me even more so psychologically.

In those moments where I cried on the floor, or stood against the wall, I hated everything. My situation, my body, and my life . . . I despised them all. This ire was emitted in ways it never should have been. My family—my loving, patient family, who stuck with me through it all—received the brunt of my anger. I by no means intentionally treated them poorly; instead, I found myself with absolutely no love or joy to share with them.

Searching deep within me, I could find nothing but a deep, dark hole that was previously my happiness. Where did it go? I truly, truly wanted to be joyful and happy, but in my heart, I was encased, engulfed by a negative, black, evil psychological and physical force. Negativity seeped out of my every pore, and I did not realize how I spoke to, or treated, my own family. Mom gently mentioned to me on several occasions to try to be nicer.

My brothers were sad, confused, and upset—not able to understand why their own sister was treating them the way she was. Where had their sister gone?

What had taken her away from them? I am filled with sadness as my reminiscence of their emotions rewinds. They never told me how they felt, but I can only imagine the internal pain they must have suffered during that time. They watched with horror as the sister they knew and loved was slowly stripped of all identification that it was actually her. Wanting to help, but unable to, my helpless brothers were left with hurting hearts, aching souls.

I rue how I made them, as well as my parents, feel . . . I crushed their spirits, and I knew it. I didn't want them to have to deal with my pain, and I wished so greatly that my suffering would not affect them. Happiness—I wanted peace and happiness for them. Sometimes, I merely desired that they give up on me, leave me; that way, I could spare them the agony of my own internal and external pain. Thinking of myself as too much of a problem, a burden, I didn't want to suck my family into it. I didn't know if I wanted to live. At times, it seemed it would be easier on my family, and me, if I did die. In fact, for a period, I yearned to die.

"Maybe it would be easier if the Lord just takes me."

"Why am I still here?"

"How do I show that I love my family . . . by living or dying?"

"I hate myself. I'm just a problem. I suck."

"Why don't they just give up on me?"

"I am closer to death than life."

"Do I give in, or claw my way back up?"

"I think . . . I'm ready to die."

The computer screen lit up Mom's face as the printer spat out paper after paper, like a toddler eating lima beans. A pink highlighter was clutched in my palm, and I sat nearby, ready to attack those freakin' papers. It was a list of side effects . . . a *lot* of side effects. We had searched for months to locate the cause of my serious issues, but it was not until my mom evoked memories from her own life that we began hiking down the correct path.

In 2004, Mom became extremely ill, and her life was nearly taken from us. A scared and helpless child, I watched my mom fight for months, barely able to move and, at times, entirely unable to. However, after three months of steady decline in her health, she pinpointed the problem. It was medication she had been taking. My mom has fibromyalgia, and amitriptyline, an anti-depressant that is used in small doses as a sleep aid, had been prescribed to treat it. Her pain makes it so that she cannot sleep, and when she doesn't sleep, her pain level goes up. When she began taking the new medication, she slept through the night for the first time in years.

However, after nearly three years of continued use, her heart began racing from it. Her doctor never suspected her medication, but Mom finally found what was killing her when she, in desperation, looked up its side effects.

Using her knowledge in this area, Mom began to investigate my medications. With the sheet of the side effects from Florinef in my hands, I began to read down the list, my pink highlighter cocked and ready for use. I was taking it for orthostatic hypotension—a result of my chemotherapy. It shocked me. The entire page had turned pink.

— Abdominal pain
— Agitation or combativeness
— Anxiety
— Back or rib pain
— Bloating
— Burning in stomach
— Chest pain or tightness
— Chills
— Confusion
— Constipation
— Difficulty swallowing
— Eye pain
— Fainting or light-headedness getting up from lying or sitting
— Fast or slow heartbeat
— Headache
— Heartburn
— Increased hunger
— Indigestion
— Irregular breathing or shortness of breath
— Irregular heartbeat

— Joint pain
— Loss of appetite
— Nausea
— Nervousness
— Pain, tenderness, swelling of feet or legs
— Pain in stomach or side, possibly radiating to the back
— Pounding in ears
— Severe dizziness
— Severe weakness in arms and legs
— Weight loss
— Unusual tiredness or weakness
— Vision changes
Less common, or rare:
    — Muscle weakness
    — Sleeplessness, trouble sleeping
    — Swelling of stomach area
    — Pressure in stomach

I had highlighted thirty-six out of eighty-nine side effects. We had found it—and I only became more astounded with more research. Medical websites included similar information.

> A wide range of psychiatric reactions including affective disorders such as irritable, euphoric, depressed and labile mood and suicidal thoughts . . . psychotic reactions, including mania, delusions, hallucinations, and aggravation of schizophrenia . . . behavioral disturbances, irritability, anxiety, sleep disturbances . . . cognitive dysfunction, including confusion and amnesia have been reported. Reactions are common and may occur in both adults and children. In adults, the frequency of severe reactions has been estimated to be 5–6%.

I was that 6 percent.

Suddenly, I realized it was not all my fault. I had a silent killer, one that eroded me physically and psychologically.

"Mushy's ditchin'!" I groaned as Mom and Dean awakened me.

It was my first day of school . . . ever. I had gradually weaned off the Florinef and was seeing a major difference in the way I felt. It turned out I would need that ounce of strength to help push through even the first day.

"Where'd *she* come from?" an agitated girl snorted to her chubby friend in Health class.

I was an alien, a freak. People looked at me strangely, and I felt as though they had X-ray vision, or a super sense of smell, that could detect I was different. I felt either watched or ignored. No one smiled at me, and they only rejected my attempts at being nice to them.

"What kind of a place is this?" I thought.

Suddenly, confusion inhabited me. Since when was disrespecting people cool? When did saying "Hi" to someone go out of style? And apparently, being a good student was so yesterday. It made me sad. Where was the happiness? The only pleasure and joy most of these kids possessed was out of sick, twisted reasons. They thought they knew everything. They thought they were grown up.

Hmm, funny, I was left thinking, "Grow up!"

Whoa, it was September 2008, and once again, my concept of time and how long I had been ill was unrealistic. My health improved with the speed of an elephant wading through peanut butter, but everyone was excited with any improvement whatsoever. Tiny signs brought flashes of hope to my everyday life. One afternoon in dance class, I found myself sweating, something I had not done in a very long time. Always having just gotten hotter and hotter, my body, at last, let me sweat. It felt so good.

On the subject of dance, it was at this time that I auditioned for the San Luis Obispo Civic Ballet's *Nutcracker*. The Civic Ballet and the Academy of Dance are connected, with the company members being the elite dancers at the studio.

They needed support cast for their show, and I recall hoping for a role such as a garland, a gingersnap . . . nothing too special. I figured they'd probably stick me in the back of the party scene, holding a tray or something, but I was entirely okay with that. I just wanted to be in it. From chemo to Civic Ballet *Nutcracker*; I was stoked.

Exhausted, I stood before a row of judgmental eyes. The audition was over, and as I stood in a straight line with a slew of sweaty classmates, roles began to be distributed immediately. Sinking lower and lower, I fought to hold myself upright as I remained in the same exact spot for what seemed like hours. I quickly glanced about the room. It looked as though every part had been chosen, all except Clara, I thought. Smiling at the two remaining girls, Kaytee and Meghan, I was positive they were the best two out of the three of us. I was right. They would be the double cast Clara, Clara A and Clara B. I was so happy for them, but where did that leave me?

"And Melinda," said Drew, the well-loved Civic Ballet's artistic director, "welcome to our studio, and we would like to offer you the part of Marie."

My jaw nearly hit the floor. Clara's sister, Marie. Next to Clara, it was one of the most important roles in the support cast. I felt honored . . . or something. Like water on concrete, it didn't really sink in. Cheers. Chaos. That's all I heard as all the girls rushed Kaytee, Meghan, and me.

An overwhelming amount of gratitude pierced my heart. It was a moment of pure joy. I truly could not grasp where I had been, what I had come through, and where I was right then. "Happiness" only brushes the surface of what I felt inside that night.

☞

More exciting news came when Dr. Dan told us that the EKG, X-ray, pulmonary function test, echocardiogram, and blood test results were all normal. In addition, the CT scan I also received that day showed that remaining scar tissue from my mass had shrunk even more. Three months—I had made it three months past treatment.

Another event to arouse my excitement was the ending of Bactrim. To refresh your memory, I shall summarize it in a few words. Giant. Bitter. Disgusting. Hell in pill form. Remember it now? At last, I would be relieved of my weekend damper. Crushing the very last tablet into a pulp, I jammed it down my throat and thanked God it was all over. I later sent a singing thank-you card to the clinic, complete with my Bactrim prescription label stuck to it—marked with a huge red "X" through it. I was so happy, I felt like either laughing or crying... I'm not sure which.

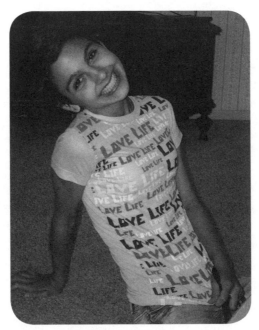

Classic Melinda.

"Let us rise up and be thankful, for if we didn't learn a lot today, at least we learned a little, and if we didn't learn a little, at least we didn't get sick, and if we got sick, at least we didn't die; so, let us all be thankful." —Buddha

TWENTY

SCHOOL HAD BECOME too much. Almost immediately, Mom and I realized that attending school for the entire day wore me out to the max. However, with Mom's requests that I cut back my hours, the school system began to show their ugly side. Soon, they had my mom jumping through rings of fire, like some sort of crazy circus act.

My school tried to jam me into one of their "selection boxes," but the problem was I didn't fit in any . . . I was too different. If we chose the "box" with me coming home after lunch, they wouldn't let me take Biology, and I really, really wanted to be able to take it. Remember what Dr. Josh told me about becoming an oncologist—I *needed* to take biology. Never before had they come across a student in my situation, and frankly, they were flustered and puzzled by me.

As Mom sent up more SOS flares, the administrators only became more stubborn. By this time, my health started to backslide; I had more and more trouble eating and depression was once again setting in. After multiple written requests for help were met with no help at all, Mom began to search elsewhere for the answer. She found that answer when her friends who work as educators told her about the 504 Plan. Casey, Lynn, Cecile, Lydia, Mary Ann, and Karl all came to my rescue, sending Mom websites to research and filling her in on my legal rights as a cancer survivor.

Not wasting any time, Mom presented a letter to my principal, requesting a 504 Plan to help me with my health struggles at school. My unresponsive counselor never told us about this option, although she is required by law to do so.

She must not have liked it when Mom found out about it through other means because, when she learned about the written request, she phoned Mom, yelling at her.

At first, she accused Mom of not letting her know how sick I was. Hello, I was *bald* when I registered for high school with her, and Mom gave her an issue of *Cottage Magazine* that told about my battle with cancer. When accusing Mom of *not* letting her know how sick I was didn't seem to work, she tried to tell Mom that I was not sick *enough*.

"Well, she *dances*."

These words slashed through Mom's heart, and she began to sob.

"If you need written documentation from Melinda's doctor stating how important dancing is to her recovery, please let me know." Mom shook with helplessness through her tears.

Immediately following the conversation, Mom called my principal, still distraught and crying. She was able to speak to Debbie Carter, the principal's very kind, compassionate secretary, and she described the verbal abuse and harassment my counselor had dumped upon her.

It was all so overwhelming to me. Sitting, watching, in my rapidly declining state, I saw Mom write what seemed like fifty letters to the school, my counselor, the principal, and the district office. She was up till the wee hours, researching and typing those letters, desperately trying to help me.

Meanwhile, I continued attending my classes as often as I could, sucking up a slew of absences when I wasn't feeling well enough to go.

"I hate this place," I thought to myself as I sat alone in the morning sun by the ceramics building that catches the mid-morning rays.

I was always freezing, constantly on the edge of what felt like hypothermia.

Those who walked by left me with their strange glances, and one girl asked, a disturbed look on her face, "Why do you sit alone?!"

It was by no means an offer to hang out with her, so I was instantly repulsed.

"I don't know," I replied.

As I watched her trudge off, I thought of how I should have replied. How could I have told her that I just *wanted* to sit alone? That I was *freezing, sick*, and *depressed*? That I just *wanted* to be *left alone*? And I hated school and, momentarily . . . life? A lump of anger and despair formed in my throat.

"Everyone just leave me *alone*!" I screamed in my head.

Just then, the bell, which had already gotten old, began to chime, and as I peeled myself off my toasty wall, I groaned. It seemed worse than death, leaving that spot to be herded, like a cow, into yet another chamber.

Stepping onto the small platform, I placed my speech before me on the podium. I carefully adjusted the microphone, smiled at the crowd of over three hundred tender expressions, and began. The spectacular Santa Barbara day was picturesque, with the sparkling shoreline clear in my vision beyond the wall of windows. Benefactors and donors of the Teddy Bear Cancer Foundation were seated at the large, elegant tables at the Biltmore Hotel's Coral Casino. I had been invited by Nikki Katz, the founder of the foundation, and Marni Rozet, the executive director, to speak and share my story. The word "no" had not even entered my mind. This was it—my opportunity to give back to them, to thank them for everything they had done.

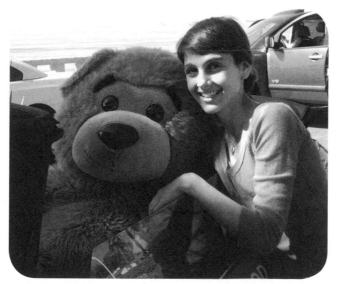

A beautiful day at the Teddy Bear Cancer Foundation Luncheon 2008.

As I gave my speech, my goal was to pierce both their hearts and their checkbooks with nothing other than the truth. I told them a story, the story of Carrie

Bear and the events of the day. Glancing up as I spoke of my anaesthesia aware-
ness mishap, I found a woman's eyes, suddenly noticing their watery, glossy
appearance. Just then, a tear escaped, slowly sliding down her cheek before a
tissue ended its journey.

When I wrote my speech, I questioned how much I should share. Pondering it
for quite some time, I decided to lay it all on the line, to give it to them straight.
Cancer *does* exist. My suffering was real, and I needed to acknowledge that. But,
something about announcing to everyone how much pain I had endured created a twist of emotions inside of me. Everything seemed gnarlier when I spoke
of it out loud, like my mind had tried to mask its severity over time. The reality
of it all hit me as I read on.

It was almost as if I was thinking, "Wow, this poor kid."

Yet, that kid was *me*. I only noticed how serious my situation was if I stepped
out of my own shoes and looked at myself from the outside. My mind had trouble grasping that *I, I* had fought, and that it was *me, me* who was the cancer survivor. Although I was able to latch onto only a tiny speck, that speck launched
an amazing feeling of pride within my soul. I guess I *had* been pretty strong, and
I guess I *had* beaten the killer of all killers.

My sense of accomplishment and pride beat even harder in my heart as I completed my speech and looked up to the group of motionless, teary-eyed figures.
There was a moment, just a moment, of silence before a roar of applause filled
the room, and the throng of people all rose to their feet. Wow. It was unbelievable. It was those few seconds that made me thankful for having had cancer. It
was exactly that which lay a molecule of worth on cancer's massive doorstep.

I was well aware that as soon as that moment ended, and cancer had sucked up
that molecule, it would once again be a matter of, "Why me?"

However, I would always have that molecule, that ounce of worth that I could
use to somewhat answer that impossible question. All of the feelings and visual
memories were forever preserved in the depths of, not my mind, but my heart,
my spirit. I consider it to be the only proper storage place for times like this.
Locked away in my soul's safe . . . I was the only one who held the combination.
The moment seemed long during it, but short after it had diminished. But I will
never forget the many impressions that day left on me.

Nikki's hug, so warm, so soft, so comforting, like the arms of an angel; she
thanked me with her love. Marni expressed her gratitude for me, gushing forth

like a ruptured water main. And my gratefulness for them created an indescribable bubble of love around us.

And final impressions: Dr. Dan leaning along the side wall with an expression so complex, I could not possibly dissect his emotions . . . Mom's words, speaking just after me, leaving every mom's heart in the room on their tables . . . a woman's gasp as Mom placed two *Beads of Courage* strands around my neck, one bright and colorful, the other entirely black, illustrating my pokes . . . a large businessman, pausing as he wrote a check to catch the tear which gently began to fall . . . my grandparents' and my dad's speechless glances, as though they'd learned something about me . . . the warm sun and cool ocean breeze hitting my face on the greatest day I had experienced in so long that I had forgotten just how long.

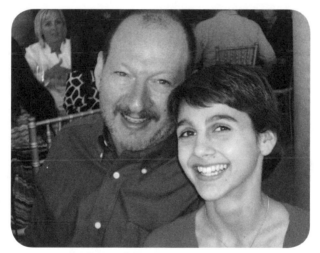

Dr. Dan and I enjoying the luncheon.

Within days of that glorious day, the third battle in my journey began. I remember it clearly. A delicious barbeque dinner sat on our kitchen table, and the entire family gathered for a weekend meal together. I picked out the squash on my plate and began eating it before I recalled seeing Mom put butter on it. Oh no. I finished it anyway, promising I would not ingest anything besides it. However, as I finished, I saw the bread leering at me from across the table, the unreal sourdough bread we toast on our grill. Oh my gosh. I wanted one piece so badly. But no, no, I couldn't have it, I just couldn't. I wasn't sure why . . . everyone else was eating it.

Remembering the promise I had made to myself, I tried to create distraction to pry the alluring bread away from me. But, I was *hungry*! Okay, okay, I would have one little piece, that wouldn't hurt me. Crunching into the crisp bread, a burst of flavor exploded in my mouth. I felt like I was going to cry . . . it tasted *so* good. Heaven. It was heaven. Barely having eaten anything all day, I suddenly lost it—I grabbed piece after piece, compulsively wolfing them down. It was as if I lost every ounce of judgment and control at that moment, and all that mattered was that bread.

Once none remained, I stumbled off to my room before collapsing in tears upon my bed. What was wrong with me? Why did I do this to myself? I was a prisoner of my own mind; I was my own Drill Sergeant. The pressure and control I shackled myself in was slowly rotting my quality of life.

"I can't live like this . . . I can't live like this," I whispered.

The very thought of the rest of my life progressing on as it was made me contemplate suicide. I couldn't go on. I wanted my life back, me back. Why was I becoming so obsessive, so controlling? I remembered back to when I first noticed how poorly I was eating. It was in Health class, the eating disorder section. There was a list of SOS signals that scared the living you-know-what out of me. It sounded just like me.

I felt insane, like my mind was possessed. It scared the hell out of me. I needed help. The constant battle in my head exhausted me beyond words, and I wanted that carefree innocence back . . . so badly that it hurt my very soul to think about it. I had become this thing, a thing I didn't recognize, a part of me that was not there before, and a something that was quickly gaining more power.

As Mom walked in to see if I was alright, I began to cry even harder. Happiness, I only wanted to be happy. Looking into Mom's eyes, I tried to be strong for her, but true despair pierced my heart. Words played hide-and-seek in my head; I finally found them and swallowed hard. How does one tell another they've lost it, gone off the deep end?

Scared of what door my words would open, I, at last, congregated my every remaining fiber of courage and said softly, "Mom . . . I want help."

She knew it was urgent. Having her degree in psychology, Mom had recognized the warning signs of an eating disorder and had suspected it all along. Frantically, she phoned the clinic, where she was able to speak with Nurse Pam. I was not present at the time, but when Mom told her of my severe troubles, my "team" at the clinic sprung into action.

Robyn located an eating disorder specialist and registered dietician in our area. Mom was relieved. The woman seemed perfect for me. I, too, felt more at ease. I wanted help, and there seemed to be hope—hope I would fully recover.

However, bad news came our way . . . the therapist did not accept our insurance, and the appointments were very, very expensive. My mom and I were overwhelmed with disappointment and heartbreak. That was it. I guess I wasn't going to get better. I guess I would either live my life in constant torture, or just eventually die. Akin to the Age of Florinef, I wasn't sure what I would rather do . . . live . . . or let God take me into His heavenly arms. One option seemed easier, more peaceful. But suddenly, on October thirteenth, we received an email from Robyn that extracted every word I knew from me, leaving me entirely speechless.

I recall driving in the car when Mom told me, "Mush . . . the Teddy Bears are going to pay for it."

The tears seeping from my eyeballs said everything for me. Never had I been so grateful to anyone, and never had I been so humbled by an experience. No words can, or will, begin to describe that moment. I felt love, thankfulness, hope, joy, and peace. Blubbering uncontrollably, I finally, fully understood what they were doing for me. They were giving me back my happiness, my love, my meaning, and my life. They were giving me . . . well, *me* back. It is, and will be, one of the greatest gifts that anyone has ever given to me. I will eternally be grateful to them and forever hold a place for the Teddy Bear Cancer Foundation in my heart.

"A gift is pure when it is given from the heart to the right person at the right time and at the right place, and when we expect nothing in return." —The Bhagavad Gita (or "Song of God")

TWENTY-ONE

THE FOLLOWING SIX months or so dragged their feet through the thick muck that was my life. Strangely, though, now that they had passed, they seemed to have pulled a Houdini, completely vanishing as a fine mist dissolves into the atmosphere. The memories are vague, yet painful, and each day seemed to mush into the next, without clear distinction. It was then that I met Heidi, a sweet, compassionate, and understanding therapist, whose thinking traveled to the depths of even my thinking. The only difference was, she could decipher those deep feelings and bring them to the surface.

That is exactly what we began to do—virtually dissect me. I learned things that few people ever discover within themselves. Feelings, motivations, and desires . . . we picked apart everything. On that tan, leather couch in Heidi's office were days of complete emotional breakdown, rebuilding, and finally, healing.

I always clutched one of the couch's soft blue pillows, gently stroking it one way and then the other. I can tell you everything about that room, for I sat there for one hour, nearly every week, for eight months. The bookshelf held a collection of eating disorder and nutrition books like you wouldn't believe. I remember staring frequently at a large blue book, although, oddly, I cannot recall the name of it. A large collection of trinkets were on display by her desk. She had the same plastic McDonald's French fries as I did. The small end table to my left was always adorned with a vase of flowers and Heidi's big, brown coffee mug, steaming with hot tea.

And when I looked directly over her right shoulder, I saw the heart, perched on a narrow ledge, that read, "Forgive yourself . . . AGAIN."

That place has become so confusing for me, happy yet sad, haunting yet hopeful. It fills my soul with gratitude, yet shatters my heart and scatters the shards. It brings me back to that time . . . the time where I had absolutely no idea I was slowly killing myself. Thinking about then and evoking memories is extremely hard and terrifying. I only now realize that, during that state, I couldn't think straight. Remembering the things I thought about and how untruthful, sick, and twisted they were, leaves me disturbed . . . very disturbed. I can recall several events in which it seemed like the end of the world. Pretty much every day seemed like the end of the world at that point, but strong memories of these occurrences continued to press my spirit as they clamored to be told.

⁓

Just after I began going to Heidi, I became increasingly stubborn about food. Not crabby stubborn, but scared stubborn.

I can still hear my mom's voice, "I want you to eat something. What do you want?"

I shook my head. I didn't want or, in my book, deserve anything. Seconds later, I saw a bowl set down next to me on the table. It was mozzarella cheese. Uh-oh.

"You need to eat it, okay?" Mom told me, as gently as she could.

"I don't care how long it takes you; you just have to eat it."

Crap. Not cheese; anything but cheese. I *couldn't*. I just couldn't eat it. I just didn't, well, actually, I couldn't eat cheese. I didn't get to . . . and that was the bottom line. As I ignored it, Mom noticed my lack of progress.

"You need to eat it. It's not going to hurt you, c'mon," she spoke truthfully, getting a little tougher with me.

That little cube of cheese was evil, and I began to agonize over consuming it. Touching it, picking it up and smelling it, playing with it—I did everything but eat it. What I was hoping was that if I put it off long enough, maybe it would get late, and I could say I was tired and wanted to go to bed. But Mom's expression told me I would be sitting there until it had disappeared down my hatch.

"Don't prolong it and torture yourself," Mom told me. "Just do it."

Picking up the hunk, I began to freak out slightly. There was one disturbing thing I would always do when food anxiety set in.

I would whisper to myself, "No, no, no, no, no, no, No!"

I yelled quietly to myself.

"I'm scared, I'm scared, no, I can't, I'm scared, no, no, can't, scared, no, no, No!"

Strange. Who, or what, was I saying "no" to? It wasn't Mom, nor any other member of my family . . . it was to me. I assume it had to do with my obsessive need for control. I was battling my own mind, trying to trick, overpower, and rule over myself.

But something tells me that it goes much deeper than all of this. I vividly remember a dark, scary feeling coming over me during those moments.

I almost had to fight it, and that is why I kept repeating, "No, no, no."

It could have been that I was saying "no," "I can't," and "I'm scared" about death, but I strongly think that I was speaking to a different thing. This thing wanted to take me over, pry away my light, my faith, my love, and my joy. It was darkness, evil, hatred, sadness, helplessness, and hopelessness, all formed into one giant ball of insanity.

I don't think I ever quite believed in a "devil" before, only Jesus my Lord . . . I do now. I used to think that insanity was kind of funny . . . I don't anymore. I believe we are all crazy to some extent, and true insanity is always within us—diminished by faith, family, and love. However, when one has been beaten down physically, spiritually, mentally, and emotionally, he or she has no reserves . . . and truly, they lose their mind. Insanity is a scary thing—I've been there.

Early that November, Mom, Dad, and I woke up one morning before dawn, to appear for outpatient surgery in a small building across the street from Cottage Hospital. It was bye-bye port. Dr. Keshen would remove the little stinker that had begun to start hurting me when I danced.

Selecting, and bringing along, a small jar from home, I asked Dr. Keshen if he could clean up my port a little and save it for me. After all, having recently read in Lance Armstrong's book that he saved his port in a jar, I immediately decided I wanted to be just like him. And so, by 4:00 that afternoon, I was lying on our living room couch, staring at my very own port in a jar on the coffee table.

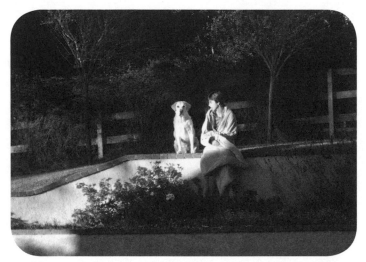

Larry and I get some fresh air and catch the evening rays after my port removal.

Having had a somewhat stressful day, I found it even more difficult when it came to food. Fasting took place before my surgery, and I found myself liking a reason not to eat. After I returned home, though, I began to play my "food games."

Upon my mom or dad asking, "What do you want to eat?" a long period of excruciating decision making would pass before I finally choked out some ideas, amid multiple repetitions of, "I don't know."

I knew I wasn't going to eat anything, but I asked for it anyway. I guess I just wanted it *that* badly, that if I wouldn't allow myself to eat it, then the next best thing was to see it, smell it. Dad brought me a potato drowned in butter . . . it must have sat there getting colder and colder for at least an hour. Mom brought a bowl of mac 'n cheese to me—a downright sin in my twisted mind. She urged me slightly, but I didn't budge. I admit that I actually pretended I had fallen asleep, that way I wouldn't have to eat it.

The games were never ending, a battle of how I could get away with not eating. I'm sorry, Mom. My mind was so, so sick, and I appreciate so deeply all the times you kept trying—more than our pitiful language can say. I am sorry I hurt you in any way, broke your heart, and if you come to me, I will sew it and mend it with my love for you.

⤳

Mom knew my weakness . . . dance. All she had to do was say the words "no" and "dance" in the same sentence, and I was jamming food down. Dance was the only thing that kept food going in me, and if not for the desire to have a speck of energy for class, I would have stopped eating altogether. Most of the time, I pulled the guilt trip on Mom, but a couple of times she kept her word, and she would not take me to dance when I didn't eat. She might as well have taken a pizza knife and stabbed my heart . . . it was the toughest love I've ever had to take.

I remember the feelings as I danced . . . exhausted, weak, unstable . . . I felt like nothing. A rack of bones; I was a dancing rack of bones. And, of course, being Little Miss Hard on Myself, I would get frustrated and upset with my body when it didn't do what I tried to make it do. Like an idiot, I wondered why, totally oblivious to the vicious cycle of me and my body not giving each other what the other wanted. One day at the studio, I recall admiring the other girls' strength.

"They get to eat," I silently whined with jealousy.

Why did I think this? I guess I thought everyone could eat but me. The disturbing thoughts continued.

"How come they get to eat, but I can't?" I asked myself.

"It's because I need to lose some weight—I'm fat . . . I need to suffer. That's what I'm meant to do . . . suffer."

⤳

Terrified of them, I counted every calorie, carb, and gram of fat in my protein bars and shakes. Everyone agreed that I needed extra protein to build my muscles back up, everyone except me. I didn't like meat; cheese and yogurt were no-no's; milk had been ruined by prednisone; and beans and pasta were repulsive. The shakes and bars were scary, but I ate them and drank them because it made my mom feel good. I had my ritual down, one soy milk shake for breakfast, an apple and a bar for lunch, and another shake after dance for dinner. Gradually, I became more and more used to my daily food items, and it became a sin to eat regular food. It was one brick wall after another in the Mind of Melinda.

The scale read seventy-nine pounds at my next clinic visit. Concern showed on the faces of Mom and Nurse Pam, but I was happy in a sick sort of way. I wanted to be seventy, sixty, fifty . . . forty—I didn't give a crud. Every moment of every day, I felt like nothing . . . physically, emotionally, and spiritually.

"Hey," I thought, "why not *be* nothing . . . look the part?"

One project, however, pulled me slightly out of my depressed state. A pen gripped in my hand, or a keyboard under my fingers, I wrote letters to a wide array of grant-giving organizations. Without even asking, I wrote to them on behalf of the Teddy Bear Cancer Foundation, told my story, and asked them to please consider giving them a grant. Immediately, the Tony Stewart Foundation responded. A lovely lady, Pam Boas, helped us with the process.

It made me feel like a person to do good for others. Really, this is the only thing that brought joy to me at that time. I possessed no personal happiness but, rather, created *my* joy by creating *others'* joy. Seeing even one smile that I had influenced was basically what I lived for. Giving, family, God, and dance . . . these are the four things that truly held my life together and made me want to keep going, keep pushing day after day.

≈

Life went on, despite everyday challenges. With assistance from Mom's incredible friends, a 504 Plan was put in place for me at school. Basically, it meant flexibility and cooperation for my unique circumstances. I would average about four periods a day: sometimes more, sometimes less. My teachers were extremely helpful and understanding, giving me assignments and work to do at home. If not for Ms. Lopez, Mr. Gracia, Ms. Jenssen, Mr. Ritchie, Mr. Long, Mrs. Long, and Mr. Hubble, I wouldn't have made it through ninth grade.

I felt sort of embarrassed I couldn't be a normal kid and go all day, and it was strange having special educational needs . . . I didn't like it. I was always worried people would think I was using my cancer as an excuse to be lazy and get out of stuff, so I tried hard to show my teachers that I did actually care. My diligence must have been apparent because I was named October's Student of the Month for the freshman class.

I even received a plaque that read, "Melinda Narchiano."

Ha, ha . . . close enough.

⤸

Thanksgiving came, and I consumed not a single bite of Gram's delicious feast. I made pies and other desserts to bring, yet sat staring at it all as I munched on my apple and protein bar. Yes, it was awkward, but I still tried to enjoy being there with my family. I have to confess, it's kind of hard when you're feeling so cruddy.

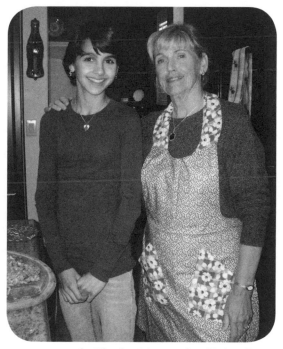

Gramma prepares the Thanksgiving meal on Turkey Day 2008.

With the holidays upon us, *Nutcracker* was kicked up a notch. I remember one rehearsal in which one of the Clara's had chicken pox. Dr. Dan had told me it could be deadly to me, and I was in freak-out mode. Thinking that, for sure, I would contract it with my weak immune system—I did not rehearse in the scene but, rather, marked it against the back wall, trying not to get in people's way. I felt stupid and different.

December eleventh was our final dress rehearsal and a Gift Performance. The rehearsal was open to none other than cancer patients and their families. Life can be filled with so much irony. Drew, our director, had asked me to say a few words to welcome the audience before curtain. As I made my way backstage with him, the other girls crowded around me.

"What are you going to say?" they all wanted to know.

Shrugging, I replied, "I don't know."

"You mean you didn't write anything? You don't have it memorized?" they asked.

"Nope," I answered with a smile.

Their eyes grew wide.

"Are you nervous?"

Chuckling, I answered with honesty, "Nope."

These were my people, and I wanted to go out there and connect with them, say something from my heart that would not lose meaning because of repetitive memorization. Standing just offstage with Drew, I could tell our nerves were on opposite ends . . . he seemed like he was a mess. Before I had too much time to think, we stepped onto stage, and the crowd applauded. Wow. There were a lot of people.

Drew talked for a minute or so, and then introduced me by calling me a "beautiful dancer who has inspired both me and the entire studio to do our best."

The smile that sprawled across my face did not begin to exhibit my feelings for what he said. Holding it together at that moment, I knew I would cry about it later. Just then, the microphone was mine. I recall thinking, as I began, that it was kind of heavy. The words just came.

As I finished, spontaneous applause broke out, and that was truly the very first time I felt like I had really done it. I had beaten cancer. The joy within me cannot be described . . . it was too beautiful for words.

Backstage once again, I found myself surrounded by teary-eyed dancers. Aw . . . I had made them all cry.

"I love you, Melinda!" Jane yelled, giving me a hug.

"You're amazing," said Alison with a smile.

"You're such an inspiration," Miranda said lovingly, and grinned.

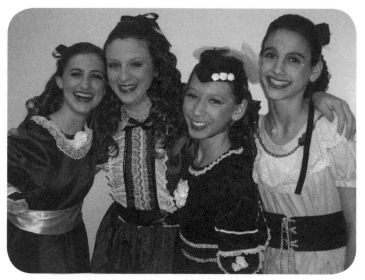

Fellow dancers Meghan, Morgan, and Amber during *Nutcracker* 2008.

Everyone had me to blame for ruining their makeup. I began to wonder, what had I done? Sure, I had beaten cancer and come to their studio less than two weeks out of treatment, but I really didn't think I was all that special. I guess I figured that all of my suffering and fighting was a part of life that I had to get through and not something that could touch other people. I never really told anyone about my cancer experience during that time because, frankly, I didn't think anyone would be interested.

However, when I was asked to speak at *Nutcracker*, and the Teddy Bear Luncheon, I thought, "Okay, I'll just tell them the truth. I won't sugarcoat anything, nor make it seem more severe than it actually was. If they really want to hear my story . . . okay. Here it goes."

That night, I was reminded that people *did* care and that they *were* interested. I have actually questioned several times, when writing this very book, if people even want to hear all of this. But I remember the many teary cast members who approached me and hugged me that night. They thought my story was special, an inspiration.

I didn't think so, and had nothing to say other than, "Thanks."

Of course, it was extremely complimentary to have those words describing me, but it put an invisible pressure on me, like I had some sort of label to live up to. But the fact that the people I touched received happiness and hope out of my story made me become okay with being "an inspiration." I didn't think I deserved it, but I was happy to accept it because it filled others with joy.

I danced that night with passion and love for life and my fellow human beings. I prayed that my cancer brothers and sisters sitting in the audience would receive even an ounce of strength to fight their own battles through watching me dance.

"Yet how hard most people work for mere dust and ashes and care, taking no thought of growing in knowledge and grace, never having time to get in sight of their own ignorance."
—John Muir

TWENTY-TWO

EMOTIONS RAN HIGH and filled my days with ups and downs. It was December eighteenth, the one-year anniversary of my diagnosis. Gratitude grasped my heart, yet the reality that nearly two years of my life had been ripped away by illness created a feeling of intense loss. At first, I imagined it was going to feel like any other day, but I soon realized that, somehow, my emotions knew the day had meaning—they felt it.

The day came and passed, going along the natural course of time progression. And as this time swiftly, yet agonizingly and slowly, moved on, my life was filled with constant psychological torment. I was now eating, but only consuming, at best, a thousand calories a day—I counted. Heidi had calculated my required amount . . . twenty-four hundred calories per day. That number scared the hell out of me.

I yearned to get healthy, both physically and psychologically, but it was so easy to give in to my mind. My two choices were either to eat, and suffer mentally, or not eat, and suffer physically. The amount of work it took to unravel and analyze every thought engulfed and burned any food that entered me. After a meal, or what I considered a meal, I would be overcome with extreme guilt, loss of control, and helplessness. Battling these emotions was draining, scary, and difficult—impossible. It was so much easier and less traumatic for me to not eat, because then my mind was pleased, not attacking me and telling me I was fat, worthless, and stupid. I felt happy when I didn't eat and had crossed over the line to where it became less upsetting to me if I didn't consume anything.

It's not fair I have to be so burdened, haunted, and scarred by it all. It's such a huge burden, responsibility. I just wanted to be a kid. Just let me *be a kid*.

Wondering why everyone wanted me to do something that made me suffer, and be unhappy, was beyond my stretch of thought. When frustrated, I would have sudden outbursts of anger that frightened me, as well as my family. Many things got thrown . . . harmless things. The worst was when I stormed into my room, grabbed the remote control for my little TV, and threw it down as hard as I could. It felt so good, that is, until I looked down to find it shattered in pieces on the floor and wondered how I would explain it all. Life was dark, grim, and I wondered how I would drag my butt through each trying day.

The feeling like it all was never going to end choked me, and so many times I told God, "Okay. I'm ready. This is too hard, Lord . . . I'm ready to go."

⤢

Christmas came, and I found myself wrapped up like a FedEx shipment, in just about every coat I owned. My family and I stood out in the blustery, frigid winds of San Simeon as we watched the elephant seals below. Who drives an hour to see seals on Christmas? Ha, ha . . . I guess we do. Watching two of the bulls fight, I began to notice how weak I felt. The cold was making me feel sick, and I hadn't eaten anything all day, because I knew we were going to go out to dinner that night. I wanted to be a normal person. Chowing a giant, seafood salad with no dressing at dinner that night, I felt guilty and promised myself, as we drove home, that I would not eat breakfast the next morning. That was my Christmas.

⤢

Throughout the course of January, I began to put on a little weight, confirmed by the rising numbers on Heidi's scale. Although I still needed to gain fifteen pounds to even register on the BMI chart, everyone said I was "doing great."

I didn't feel any better, so I thought, "Why have the added weight? It just makes me fat, ugly, and stupid."

Late-night sit-up sessions and running suddenly became an obsession. Anxiety would permeate me if one day went by without some type of rigorous exercise.

I didn't do it because I wanted J-Lo's body, or something stupid like that. I just wanted so badly to feel good about myself. My desire for worth was so intense that I would have done nearly anything to be happy with myself, have a sense of purpose, and feel that I mattered.

&

But it was *him* ... it was *him* who beat me down. I say "him" because that's exactly what it was like: two separate people, two different voices. Heidi explained it in a way that made so much sense. She explained that my "healthy voice" was the real me, the Melinda that is funny, joyful, carefree, and wants to heal. Going on, she described my "unhealthy voice" as a liar, a deceiver who tricked me into thinking my life didn't matter and who wanted to make me suffer.

After using the phrase "unhealthy voice" for quite some time, I invented a new name for him ... "Mr. Stupid." I believe he slowly formed with each traumatic event that I went through. Staying so strong at the time, my emotions slowly formed a dark psychological mass in place of my physical mass. My extreme sensitivity did not help the matter; it only created deeper crevasses that Heidi had to excavate.

Seeing, hearing, smelling, and tasting only skim the surface of my senses ... I *feel* things—everything. My memories are feelings, sometimes associated with something like a color or a shape. I've always found comfort in familiar things and rituals. They don't give me that strange new feeling. So, after over a year of constant new "feelings" that I could not identify and put in their place, I began to lose it. But again, that is only one tiny, narrow side of what caused my eating disorder.

&

Walking with a crowd of girls into the huge, bright dance studio, I was overcome with emotion. I was actually *there* ... at the San Francisco Ballet. I had spent the last two days auditioning in the area for summer ballet intensive programs. Basically, they are rigorous training summer camps for dancers. The Pacific Northwest Ballet and Walnut Hill sessions had gone fairly well, and I began to observe the other girls as I stretched out before the Boston Ballet audition.

Wow. They were good . . . *freaky* good. Uh-oh. Suddenly I realized something, and my heart fell to my, well, on second thought, we won't go there. I saw a sea of black camisole leotards and stared wide-eyed, before looking down at mine. *Bright red halter*. Oops. In pre-audition excitement, I had mixed up the requirements of two of the auditions. One recommended wearing a bright color to stand out, while the other was strictly black camisole.

Yeeaahh . . . suddenly I didn't trust myself anymore. The looks I received added stress to my already stressful situation. I got up, standing still for a moment, working up the courage to go up to teachers and leaders of the Boston Ballet and apologize for my leotard.

"They're gonna think I'm the stupidest thing on Earth," I thought, as I stepped to face them.

I don't even remember exactly what I said . . . something about how sorry I was that I had gotten confused.

I probably looked like a suck-up, and as I walked away pinning a number to my clown costume, I thought, "@#*&! They're going to be watching me the *entire* time."

Their eyes burned a hole in the back of me; it was so uncomfortable. The girls were then lined up at the *barre* in numerical order. It just so happened that I ended up in the far left, back corner, with all the dance bags. Ugh. But, oh well, at least I knew they could see me all the way from a different freakin' state!

After *barre* work, we did center combinations in groups. We would all learn the combos together in one huge group, so there I was, in the exact, dead center of the crowd of seventy. I was the red bull's-eye on a black dartboard. But, as the audition's pianist began to play the tender, graceful, yet powerful adagio music, and I began to dance to it, something melted in my heart. Each step felt so good . . . heavenly. And the music, oh the music, it pierced my very spirit as I let it move my body and soul as one.

Seeing the attentive, judging eyes in my peripheral vision, I suddenly didn't care about anyone else . . . it was my moment, and no one could take that away from me. All of my accomplishments, everything I held dear in my heart—no one could take it away. Discovering tears in my eyes as I finished with only the slightest wobble, I held the flood back. I could have easily erupted into sobs and broken down right then . . . I was so happy.

The judges never looked to me, or began whispering to one another, or wrote anything down, but I didn't care one bit. They could have screamed in my face that I was the crappiest dancer on the planet and a disgrace to the dance world and I would have been just fine with that. It wasn't about extending my leg up to my ear, or having incredible turn out, or having an arch like a horseshoe. No, what mattered was *dance*. When I moved, whether it was beautiful or the ugliest thing on the planet, I felt nothing but joy. Every single emotion that polluted me somehow transformed into one giant wad of love, fire, and happiness. In the car on the way home, I retold the story, through my tears of joy, explaining to Mom how I felt.

"And it was like, here I am!" I shouted enthusiastically.

"Love me in my red leotard, hair not long enough for a bun, and gushing with tears!"

You know, I think you kind of have to be screwed up to be a really great dancer. One can be normal and just have natural ability, or one can dance with that inner pain that somehow morphs into passion and unbelievable grace with each movement. It's beautiful, touching, breathtaking.

Back at the clinic, I watched from my tabletop perch as Dr. Dan assumed the "mind probe" position. The mind probe was the name I had creatively thought of for his thinking pose. With eyes shut, and squeezed as tightly as they could possibly be, Dr. Dan bowed his head and gently pinched the bridge of his nose. Ooo . . . it was a good one. In silence, I waited . . . and observed his style of . . . let's say . . . meditation that was rather . . . well . . . unique.

After taking a giant, deep, lung-filling breath, he switched positions. With his hand raised, as if he was taking an oath or worshiping something, Dr. Dan kept his eyes glued shut. Maybe he was calling upon some oncology god. I tried not to giggle for fear of distracting him from his method of concentration and, I'm sure, composure. A long, cleansing exhale emerged from deep within him, and after lowering his hand, he flipped his wrist palm up, as if presenting something to me. Then, he opened his eyes and smiled.

I have to admit, I would sometimes imitate him.

"Mind probe . . . ," I would say, emulating his nose pinch.

"Praise," I would call out before switching over poses.

"Present," I continued, my palm outstretched.

"Mind probe . . . praise . . . present."

"Mind probe . . . praise . . . present."

Repeating it over and over, I would do one, then the other, one, and then the other. It provided many needed laughs and lots of long car trip entertainment.

But anyway, back to my story. I had received a CT scan that day, and Dr. Dan reported that the mass had shrunk *even more*. He explained that something would always be in my chest in the form of scar tissue, but as the cancer cells within this tissue died, the mass sort of "deflated." Whoa. That was cool. Deflation rocks. Dr. Dan then examined me, feeling the lymph nodes in my neck.

He always asked, "Pain, pain, pain?" as I struggled to control my ticklishness.

"Pain, pain, pain? Pain, pain, pain?"

Upon observing my legs, he found multiple bruises. I could see the slight look of concern on his face. Unexplained bruising meant internal bleeding . . . not good.

Asking if I knew what they were from, I excitedly answered, "Dance!"

"Dance?!"

Dr. Dan's eyes shifted from my bruises to me.

"Since when is dance a contact sport?" he sputtered.

February fourteenth, Valentine's Day, started out to be a very hard, horrible, end-of-the-world day. However, I received a surprise during my third period Nipomo High School Dance Company class at school. In walked a man followed by two other men and a woman, all clad in red and white striped vests. Aw . . . it was a barbershop quartet. Class stopped. Everyone was confused. What was going on?

A strange feeling, almost a tickle, was in my stomach, or was it my heart? Suddenly, I heard my name, and the man stepped forward and placed a red flower in my hands. Of course, I began to cry. It was Darrell, a man from Gloria Dei Church, where my dad plays the piano. He had told my mom that he wanted to sing to me on Valentine's Day with his barbershop quartet, and that is exactly what they began to do.

The entire class stood in awe as I clutched my flower and listened to their beautiful, harmonious songs, my face turning from white, to pink, to red with each one of my tears. They had no idea how much I needed love, hope, and joy that day. They brought that to me, and I will forever be grateful and always remember how, suddenly, I went from the lowest of lows to the highest of highs.

Another event happened at school, although this one was less than fortunate. People were mean. Several run-ins with students began to affect me, scar me. One kid in my Biology class upset me so greatly that I cried the whole way home. From previous inquiries about my absences he knew that I had fought cancer. One day, when I returned after missing multiple classes, he questioned me. "Where have you been? Sick?"

I nodded.

"Man! I wish I could just go home all the time!"

Those words ignited a fire inside of me. I was furious.

"No you don't," I said, remaining calm despite my anger.

"Yeah, I do; that must be nice," he shot back.

I remained stubborn. "Trust me, you don't," I insisted before turning a cold shoulder to him.

Words screamed in my head.

"You @#*&! If only you knew how much I suffered, and how much I would *love* to be able to make it through even *one* day without feeling like crud! And don't you think for one second that I use my illness to get out of school! I would kill to be *able* to come to school! I'm sitting here right now, feeling like %#@*! Maybe if I puke in your face you'll believe that I *am* sick! You stay home with a cold! A *cold*! I had *cancer* . . . . &*#@ *cancer*! You get to feel good! You get to be healthy! I would give anything, *anything*, to feel that way for one millisecond. I would pour my guts out on this table right now, just to know what it feels like. I don't even *&#@ remember what it feels like!"

Tears welled up in my eyes. I couldn't focus, and my rage blurred every word that Mr. Ritchie spoke. I just wanted people to believe me . . . that's all.

"Bitterness is like cancer. It eats upon the host. But anger is like fire. It burns it all clean." —Maya Angelou

TWENTY-THREE

AT THIS TIME, about mid-February, I began to write this very book. A spiral notebook became an extension of my hand, and I was never seen at school without it tucked under my arm.

"Why are you always doing homework?" kids would ask.

"I'm not," I would reply. "I'm writing a book."

You can probably imagine the skeptical glances I was thrown. I want to let those people know, right now, that I forgive them, and I'll still gladly sign a copy for them.

To be honest, I never wrote with an ending point, I just wrote . . . wrote about my life and what happened to me. I was the weird girl, sitting in the sun at break with twelve layers of clothes on, doing "homework." Diligently, during wasted classroom time, which there's a lot of, I hopped from that day's lesson to my notepad and back. Something felt good when I wrote. People could think whatever they wanted to think, but I had something incredible in that little notebook . . . my story. No one could take that away from me.

The day sucked. It was not even ten in the morning, and it *sucked*. In some sort of previous-night atoning of "food sins," I did not eat breakfast. Allowing myself one dried piece of mango mid-morning, I fell into a sudden binge. After what seemed like a pound of mangoes, my stomach and entire digestive system shrieked at me. With tears rolling down my cheeks, out of physical pain and emotional rue, I hopped into the car.

I was determined to go and see Lance. That's right, Lance . . . Lance Armstrong. As Mom and I entered the quaint, Danish village town of Solvang, about forty-five minutes from home, we eyed the entire bicycling community out in full force to watch the Tour of California Time Trials. I held in my hands my port jar as we strolled through the crowds, taking in the sights. It was a spectacle.

"We're gonna get Lance to sign my port jar!" I had joked with Mom the whole drive.

After asking several people where Lance's team camp was, we must have walked five miles, with several wrong directions and more searching. At last, by chance, we stumbled upon it. A huge mass of fans had already grown around it, like moss on a wet rock. We squeezed in, ending up in the dead center of the pushing and unruly crowd. It was intense, and the temperature rose with the heat of a million bodies. Whew, I think I was breaking a sweat—we must have stood there over an hour.

Suddenly, a roar from the crowd told me that Lance had emerged from the camper. Craning my neck, I finally spotted him. Wow. This was unreal. I couldn't believe where I was and who I was looking at. We watched as he mounted his stationary bike and began to warm up. His strength amazed me. I wanted a quarter of it, an eighth of it—a *hundredth* of it.

Trying to move in closer, I found I was stuck, pinned on all four sides. I could see Lance through a tiny slit, but that was good enough for me. He then dismounted and made his way over to the waiting fans. The ocean of people surged, pushing to the front. I held on for the ride. After signing only one auto-graph, Lance grabbed his bike and was off through a small opening in the bar-rier. The crowd ran after him, rushing to the starting area to watch him begin his time trial.

Just then, I realized no one stood around me—not even one person. And the front, well, there was no "front," it was empty. I stepped forward . . . we were going to wait right there until he got back. And come back he did, bringing the mass of people with him. I held my spot, smooshed against the orange-colored steel barriers. A TV camera stood to my left, and after disappearing into the camper for a few minutes after his time trial, Lance returned.

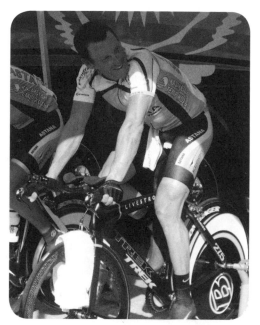

Lance warms up before his time trial.

Making his way around the crowd, he began to sign a few things. Holding my port in the jar, I began to wave it in the air as he came closer and closer. He neared where I was . . . oh my gosh. Stopping at the camera, he began to be interviewed, not even two feet away from me. We were basically face to face, and I joked that I was so close I could have reached out and picked his nose for him.

I made my jar visible, propping it up on top of the barrier. A reporter, also to my left, began asking questions, and as Lance answered, I saw him peeking at my port in the jar. He knew what it was; I can almost guarantee it. As he glanced at it five or six times throughout the interview, I felt my heart skipping beats . . . this was unbelievable. The interview ended, and I found myself handing my port over to Mr. Lance Armstrong.

"What's this?" he asked.

"Well," I replied over the noise of the crowd, "I'm a survivor too, and I saved my port in a jar, just like you did!"

He chuckled, and I felt an instant kinship with him. He had been there.

"Is here fine?" he asked, pointing to a spot on the jar.

He could have signed a dirt clod and I would have been thrilled.

"Yeah," I answered, "anywhere."

With big, beautiful, graceful sweeps of his Sharpie, Lance autographed my jar.

I was barely able to squeak out a "Thank you so much" before the overeager crowd demanded more signatures.

Holding it high above the heads of others, and careful not to smudge it, I wound through the maze of people and finally popped out into the open. It was things like this that kept me going. I had wanted to die that morning, but suddenly, life was the best thing that ever happened to me. Staring at what I held in my hands, I felt weightless. That didn't just happen ... but it did.

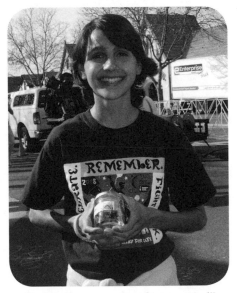

"Lance Armstrong signed my port jar!"
"Your what?!"

It helped me to have my mind focused on something, keeping me away from that "what now?" post-cancer feeling. Giggling at the silly St. Patrick's Day parade rolling by, Mom and I waited to be called in for our appointment at California

& Main. I examined the exquisite dresses in the window display . . . yes, it was a dress shop well known for those seeking a special and unique gown.

Okay, you're probably wondering, "What did *she* need a dress for?"

So, here's the story. One typical March day, I went out and got the mail as I usually do.

I found an envelope addressed to me that read, "Cities of America, Inc."

Ripping it open, I began skimming the letter. It was an offer to compete in the Miss Jr. Teen Santa Barbara Pageant.

"Ha, me—in a pageant," I instinctively thought, before handing it over to Mom.

Discussing the matter, I began to warm up to the idea. From what I had read, it didn't seem like a weird pageant, it sounded kind of . . . well . . . cool.

"You know," Mom told me, "this might be an opportunity that God is giving you."

"Yeah," I responded, "I was thinking that too."

We both had a funny feeling staring at that envelope. There would be an information session in Santa Barbara soon. Mom and I set the letter aside, determining that we would see how I felt that day and maybe take a drive down.

Well, the Sunday information session day came, and a beautiful, sunshiny day greeted us. It just so happened I needed distractions and a getaway, and before long, we were sitting among what seemed like hundreds of girls and their moms in the ballroom of the Fess Parker Double Tree Resort. I think I laughed the entire time. After filling out a form, taking a Polaroid, and listening to a woman's pageant speech, my row was escorted into the hall and lined up against the wall. We would be interviewed by one of the three judges at the individual tables before us.

Looking up and down the line, I observed what the other girls were wearing. The nervous girls were all clothed in tight, professional-looking women's suits, horribly uncomfortable shoes, and those thick waist belts that I never quite understood the purpose of. I'm all about comfort. In a pink skirt, some shirt I can't remember, and my Converses that I probably should have washed, I felt a little out of place. Something about me, at that point in my life, made me not care, though, not give a darn about what people thought of me. As I sat down to be interviewed, it is not that I didn't give my best effort; I just didn't try to be something, or someone, I wasn't.

I didn't give a crud if the woman laughed in my face, shouting, "*You*?! *You* want to be in a pageant? You actually think you can win a pageant?!"

Not believing I was pageant material, I threw myself out there as Melinda, not some high-strung, stuck-up beauty queen with a cheesy, fake smile and unnaturally white teeth. But anyway, a short time passed before we received a letter in the mail. I had been accepted to compete. I sort of thought I would make it in, but at the same time, I kind of didn't think I would.

❧

Suddenly realizing that I needed a dress, heels, and sponsors, several loving people came to my aid. Mr. Travis Wilson, who our friends from the Teddy Bear Cancer Foundation contacted, generously chose to be a sponsor. Also, The Floor Connection, owned by Mom's cousin Lory and her husband, Jim, stepped up to the plate in a heartbeat. And Priscilla, incredible Priscilla, who had bought the wig for me, made an unbelievable deposit into the Melinda fund.

She told me, "Go and find the perfect dress . . . one that makes you feel like a princess."

And that is exactly what I felt like as I emerged from the dressing room in a long, strapless ball gown. Our dear friend, Vicki, who I mentioned in my chemo days, met us there, and both she and Mom gasped as I stepped before a giant wall mirror. Wow. Fading from deep purple at the top, to light lavender at the bottom, the dress's intricate beadwork was breathtaking. It was the one. I had wondered, upon arriving, how I would possibly choose a dress among the hundreds and hundreds hanging everywhere in the small shop. As I tried on each gown they brought to me, none stood out as much as the purple one. I couldn't stop looking at it. A size 2. The man who owned the store pinched the excess fabric, showing me what it would look like after it was taken in. It would fit like a glove. With my eyes fixed on my reflection, I felt beautiful, in every way imaginable, for the first time in a long, long time.

❧

This time, my interview wardrobe was stepped up. In a bright yellow dress, black sweater, and black high heels—yes, *me* . . . in heels—I waited my turn. I was on deck. Smiling at the girl next to me, I concluded she was as fake as Donald Trump's hair . . . her smile . . . her demeanor . . . everything.

"Whoa girl," I thought to myself, "just chill . . . you're trying *way* too hard."

Before another thought could hatch in my mind, I was called into yet another Fess Parker Double Tree ballroom. How many were there? The maze of them confused me.

"Hi," I greeted the row of judges, "I'm Melinda Marchiano, and I'm contestant number fifty-seven."

We had been told what we had to say when walking in, and as I sat down in front of them wearing a huge smile, just about everything I had learned from the training session the week before flew out the window.

"Now, there are three options of ways to sit for your interview," I remember Brian, our very "interesting" training dude, stating while he demonstrated.

Bologna! I didn't need to sit a certain way for them to like me. And plus, if they did give me a bad score for sitting in "option 4 position," then it wasn't the type of pageant I wanted to be a part of.

"Make sure you have eye contact," Brian's voice echoed in my head.

What? Like I wasn't going to look at the people I was talking to?! I concluded that I'd forget Brian's less-than-helpful hints. Phew. I felt better already. The other girls waiting in the hall had been stressing over remembering every little thing . . . poor things. The questions began—normal, everyday, get-to-know-you questions.

"Who is your favorite celebrity?" I recall one woman inquiring.

"Lance Armstrong," I replied, pointing to the Livestrong bracelet around my wrist.

"I fought cancer last year, so he's a big inspiration to me."

I wanted them to know I had battled cancer because that was now a part of who I was. Yet, at the same time, I had wondered how to go about doing it—I did not want my experience to give me an unfair advantage over others.

I wanted to get as far as I could being me, just me, and that is exactly what the judges received after asking, "What's your favorite animal?"

"Hmm," I thought out loud. "I like monkeys. And oh, squirrels! I like squirrels because they're cute!"

The foursome laughed at my reply. A man, the youngest judge, then began to speak. There was something about him that made me feel very comfortable.

"Watch a movie, read a book, or write a book . . . which would you rather do?" he asked, his intense eyes looking straight through me.

"Well, actually," I responded truthfully, "I *am* writing a book. So, write a book!"

I could see the curiosity within him as he questioned me further.

"Yes, it's about my experience with cancer," I told him.

Pondering my answer, some kind of wheels were obviously turning in his head, it seemed to me. Then, just as quickly as it began, the interview ended. I shook hands all around, thanked them for their time, and made my way out the door. As I made for the exit, I could feel the one male judge watching me. There was something familiar, yet different, and unique about him. He seemed important, successful. Hmm.

The following day was the pageant. We stayed Friday night, after my personal interview, at the same hotel the Teddy Bears had previously provided for us during my treatment. Rehearsal was the next morning. As Mom and I entered the Lobero Theater's backstage area, a man handed me my contestant number to pin on. The theater had to be, like, a bajillion years old, but it was pretty neat. Pictures and autographs lined the walls as we followed the signs to find the dressing room.

Kissing Mom good-bye, I suddenly realized that it was actually happening. Waiting for the curtain to rise for my group's Casual Wear portion of the pageant, I adjusted my ballet skirt and pulled up my striped leg warmers. They encouraged us to be ourselves in the Casual Wear Competition, suggesting we wear what we wear "daily," or what we like to do. In full ballet attire, I suddenly had an idea . . . I was going to go for it. I decided that, instead of doing a pivot in the walk Brian had taught us, I would do a half-*relevé* turn on *pointe*. As I practiced backstage, the other girls looked concerned.

"Are you really going to do that?" they asked, as if they were shocked I would take such a risk.

"Yeah," I answered simply.

"Are you nervous?" one contestant questioned me, looking quite frightened herself.

"No," I replied, practicing one last time.

The only butterflies fluttering within me were butterflies of excitement. Just then, the curtain rose, and the hot stage lights hit my face as I tried not to squint.

⌒

Before I knew it, the stage was mine . . . time for my walk. I don't know what psychotic train hit me, but at that moment, I began to walk forward; not normally, but as though I was in ballet class. I guess it was just an instinct. Completing my walk, I hit my mark and rose up onto my *pointes*. My heart plunged as I heard a quiet gasp from the audience before a roar of applause.

Assuming my place back in line, it was not long before I was downstairs changing into my gown, trying not to let it touch the dirty, dusty, indistinguishable production equipment that also occupied the dressing room area. There was a lot of waiting before the curtain rose for the Formal Wear Competition. There must have been thousands of dollars of dresses lined up as we each stepped forward to answer our age division's question.

Our question was, "What one word best describes you?"

I had thought about it backstage while I waited. My initial decision had been "passionate," but I had heard a girl in a previous group use it. I mused before coming to terms with "determined." My nerves jumped for the first time when the really fake girl I met at the interview spoke.

"I'm determined because . . ."

Crud. What now? What one word describes me and absolutely no one else? What will no one choose? Hiding my disappointment behind a smile, the lightbulb suddenly clicked on.

"Courageous."

I was "courageous."

I was thoroughly confident that no one would say anything close to that. As I stepped up, hit my mark, and recited my name and contestant number, the emcee repeated the question and waited for my answer.

"What one word describes you, and why?"

"I believe courageous describes me," I explained. "I had cancer last year. I beat it, now I'm here, and I am just so thrilled."

Cheers erupted, and I felt amazing as I took my walk to the edge of the stage, twirled, and began to walk again. Beautiful ... incredible ... is how I felt at that moment. Just like a princess ... I felt just like a princess.

There was *more* waiting and more waiting and, yep, you guessed it, more waiting before all of the contestants were herded onto the stage. It was time to announce Miss Photogenic, Miss Congeniality, and the top ten girls from all four age divisions. I was in the Jr. Teen Division, and stood among my fellow Jr. Teens as Miss Photogenic was crowned. She was a little one, very cute, with a contagious smile.

"And now, we are going to announce Miss Congeniality 2009," the emcee shouted enthusiastically.

I was curious to see who it would be. All of the girls had cast a vote.

"Contestant number ... fifty-seven, Melinda Marchiano! Congratulations!"

Like an idiot, I almost had to double-check my number. That was *me*! I thought it was hysterical and laughed and smiled as a trophy, ten times larger than any basketball trophy I've ever received, was placed in my hands. I immediately thought of the pageant movie, *Miss Congeniality*, and could not believe that sort of stuff actually happened to people. The pageant world was so new to me; I didn't know it really existed, what went on, or how *it felt*. I did now.

Resuming my position in the crowd, I received congratulations and smiles from some, snorts and envy from others—vicious, pageant girls.

I thought, "Go ahead! Sabotage me!"

I witnessed one girl turn green with jealousy as I was announced for the top ten Jr. Teen contestants. It's very awkward dealing with envious people, because really, it's their own problem. I just remained gracious and happy with how far I had gotten. The top ten girls all remained outside, in the theater's back area, while the judges deliberated. We would go in one more time, group by group, and select a card that held our mystery, final question. It seemed the girls were in a tizzy over not knowing what they would be asked.

I thought to myself, "Hey! It's a *question*. All you have to do is answer it truthfully."

And that is exactly what I did as I was escorted by my hand to the front and read my mystery card.

"What family values do you have?" it asked.

Repeating the question over in my head, I let the words begin to flow out. I said something about respect, love, and helping each other through tough times. To be truthful, I don't remember my mouth moving, it felt more like my heart.

Finishing up, I was saluted with a round of applause. I saw my mom on the very end of a row and smiled toward her. My high heels began to kill me as we waited for what seemed like an eternity. However, the cool evening air in the courtyard refreshed me . . . it had been like a furnace in that place. It was interesting, hearing the girls' comments.

"If I don't win this thing, I'm going to hear about it from my mom the whole way home."

Sheesh. I felt bad for her. My mom would love me to death if I tripped on my dress, fell off the stage, and came in last. My eavesdropping continued until we were, at last, called back on stage. The table of tall trophies glittered from behind the curtain to my left.

"It would be cool if I got one, but it is fine if I don't . . . I'll still be happy," I remember thinking.

I stood with a huge, joyful smile on my face, as the 4th, 3rd, 2nd, and 1st runners-up were announced.

"Oh well," I thought at first, before getting a slight sensation within me.

Could it be me? It has always seemed to me that when someone is expecting something, it doesn't happen, and when someone isn't expecting something, that "something" happens. It's true.

"Contestant number . . . fifty-seven, Melinda Marchiano!" the emcee yelled, as I gasped, wide-eyed.

In a blur, I stumbled forward, stopping as a crown and sash were placed on me. I was in awe. A nearly three-foot-tall, sparkling, red and gold trophy was set next to me, and I raised it up in my arms for a waiting photographer.

After cuing me for my victory walk, the emcee announced, "Here she is, taking the stage for the first time as your new Miss Jr. Teen Santa Barbara, 2009!"

Waving to the crowd, I felt nothing but happiness. The feeling I had within my spirit cannot be described, nor will it even be able to be re-created. It was something I had never felt before . . . a bursting of gratitude, love, and who knows what else, all displayed in one smile and two twinkling eyes.

Exactly one year before, I had been in the hospital getting my last chemo pumped into me. I had worn a plastic crown . . . now I had a real one. My make-shift, crepe paper sash had also transformed. The maraca in my hand was now a trophy, and instead of a dirty, ugly, diamond-print hospital gown, I was wearing a ball gown—a beautiful, purple, beaded ball gown. And once again, life's irony amazed me.

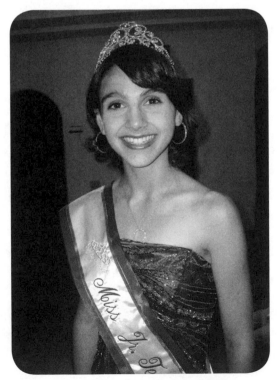

Miss Jr. Teen Santa Barbara 2009.

To top off the magical night, one of the judges approached me, a business card outstretched in his hand.

It read, "Matt Hackney."

He was the judge who had displayed a great interest in my writing during the Personal Interview. Standing before me in his white suit and shoulder-length hair, he, interestingly, resembled Jesus. I was speechless when I heard the words he spoke.

"Melinda, I would like to help you publish your book."

And, just like that, the broken pieces of my heart were glued back together.

"And in the end, it's not the years in your life that count.
It's the life in your years." —Abraham Lincoln

TWENTY-FOUR

AFTER REACHING the highest of highs I had risen to in a good year and a half, it is scary to remember just how quickly things began to spiral downward. A free fall. I was in a free fall.

The strength I needed to battle and cope with my physical and psychological problems every single . . . well, second, really began to take a toll on me emotionally. I couldn't do it . . . it was too hard, too painful, in some twisted mental way. I couldn't let myself have what I wanted, whether it be food, rest . . . whatever. Realizing that I was unknowingly, and unintentionally, tricking my mom and others into thinking I ate more than I did, I suddenly felt ashamed of myself.

I was staying in my comfort zone, where I would eat barely anything, but I would tell Mom, "I ate."

I would throw away food Mom would give me that I considered "a sin" in my mind. Recalling the feelings I had as I stuffed food into the bottom of our trash can is so strange now. It was one night, out in our spa, that I broke down and cried to her.

"Mom, I don't want to trick you! I love you, and I'm sorry! I don't mean to, I just do it, and it scares me! I'm sorry! I love you so much!"

I was afraid that my eating disorder was slowly pulling us apart. It was as if, at this time, I became scared by the natural flow of eating a little bit more and more, of stimulating recovery.

"I ate! Why do I want more food? No! I *already* ate!"

It never quite occurred to me that what I was eating wasn't enough. This lack of food sometimes caused daily binges. I would allow myself a bite of something, after determining that I "deserved it," knowing in my mind that, upon that first bite, I would become uncontrollable. However, I tried so hard to control myself that it hurt, as my hand, involuntarily, kept grabbing at food.

There was this sudden rush I would get, like my blood pressure was instantaneously going from zero to one thousand. It felt so good; I couldn't stop. Eating more and more and more, it seemed I never became full and only desired food even more with each bite. The only cue that signaled the end of the Melinda Binges was a physical stomach pain or general sick feeling. It was then that the extreme, remorseful breakdown would occur—it was a never-ending cycle.

This reminds me of one traumatic evening, which still haunts my mind. It had been a typical day . . . lack of food, and a night of wandering around the kitchen, starving, looking for something that I "deserved." Opening the fridge, I was met by my worst enemy at the time . . . dessert. I had baked a cheesecake.

"*@$%!" I thought, staring at the horrible, mean, taunting cake.

It looked so good, but I knew if I was to take one teeny, tiny crumb—that would start a cheesecake face-stuffing session. I was so afraid of losing control and had absolutely no trust that I would eat a normal amount. I lifted the plastic wrap silently and smelled it. That's what I did when I "couldn't have" something I wanted. Closing the fridge, I began to walk away . . . I didn't "need" cheesecake. But just as I thought that, my mind shouted thoughts at me with light speed.

"But you *want* some!"

"You need to let yourself have what you want!"

"You're fat! You don't need cheesecake!"

"How do you ever expect to get better if you don't try?!"

"You're just going to eat the whole thing, like a pig!"

I weighed seventy-nine pounds. The mental torture of "not being able" to have what I wanted, and what my mind would do to me if I *did* have some, paralyzed me.

Frustrated and overwhelmed, I thought, "Screw it. I'm gonna have what I want."

And as I squeezed the cheesecake out of the fridge and took my first bite, I almost felt proud for a moment, proud that I had overcome my own personal barrier. But then, suddenly, I became terrified. It was so smooth, so rich . . . like nothing I had tasted in months.

You can probably guess what happened next. Control steadily slipped from my slippery hands and fell in a splat on the kitchen floor. I don't recall how long I stood there, repeatedly stuffing my face with bite after bite, barely able to take a breath in between. The red light came on to stop me when I began to feel sick, and I finally set down my fork.

Oh my gosh. A dark, deep, demonic regret pierced my very soul. I wanted to die at that moment. Angry, helpless sobs spurted out of me, and I picked up my fork once again. I had a plan . . . I was going to eat until I threw up. Continuing my binge, I ate until it became hard to swallow, and I was nearly gagging on each bite. Shoving the cake back into the fridge, I walked over and stood, hovering over the kitchen sink . . . waiting . . . waiting.

I was so mad at myself for allowing myself to have even a single crumb. It was official in my mind: I was a pig . . . fat . . . stupid . . . psychotic . . . and sick. It was the end . . . I was sure of it. Still waiting, I became frustrated I was not throwing up, and instead of going back for more, I started jumping around like a nut, trying to make myself sick.

I want you all to know that I was not me when I did this sort of thing. I didn't decide to do what I did. My mind made its own decisions, forcing my body to go along with it. I lived in fear that my mind would make me do something I didn't want to do. Listening to my sick mind was exhausting to the real me, yet if I didn't listen, it would make me feel worthless . . . entirely worthless.

As I ran over to the sink after my jumping outbreak, still nothing would come. Crying like a slave being beaten, I took my finger and placed it in my mouth. I had never made myself throw up before . . . I was scared, mortified actually. I didn't want to do it, but I just wanted to *feel good* and please my mind. Sticking my finger back further, I became more frightened.

"I can't. I can't," I said to myself, thinking about my future.

I knew if I made myself throw up, even one time . . . that would be it . . . I would be hooked. That would probably do it, do me in . . . kill me. Suddenly, I thought of my family and especially my mom. I love them too much. I couldn't leave them, break their hearts like that.

"I don't want to die! I don't want to die!" I sobbed, taking my finger out of my mouth and collapsing in a nearby doorway.

I wanted to be healthy and normal so badly, but at that moment, it seemed so much easier to listen to my twisted, evil mind, throw up, stop eating, and, well . . . die. The worst thing we can possibly have in life is no hope. Without hope, we drown in darkness and suffocate as if the very devil has possessed us. That is exactly the way I felt that night.

꩜

Along with my extreme psychological problems were many physical issues as well. My digestive system had become so whacked-out that I strongly desired to just rip it out altogether. Turns out, it was another Melinda vs. Drug War. Miralax, the "harmless" powder I drank in liquid every day, had formed mini-sandbars in my intestines, blocking everything it was supposed to *unblock*. I stopped taking it immediately and instantly felt improvements. Yeah—Miralax—not such a "Mira"-cle for me. Anger boiled inside of me for all the times dance class had been ruined, entirely un-enjoyable because of my intestinal problems. At many times, it was almost too painful to move, let alone dance. I concluded that the white powder was evil, and I swore that no other drugs would ever pass my lips, if I could help it.

꩜

On the subject of dance, I began to need it more and more, it being my only source of happiness as I spiraled downward mentally and physically. I remember wondering, as Mom and I drove to San Luis for my last before-break class, how I was going to make it through the one week of Spring Break without dance. It had been an end-of-the-world-day, and, of all the times I needed dance the most, it was then. I looked forward to putting every ounce of my strength and emotions into moving until I came to that happy place . . . numb physically and mentally, but still going for it.

But suddenly, as we turned into the cul-de-sac usually lined with cars, I knew something was wrong. It was empty . . . it was all empty. With my life in such disarray, I had gotten confused. The break started *that day*. In one instant, I was full-on sobbing, with my heart cut out and mangled on the dashboard. I *needed* dance so badly that day, and I truly thought I would die without it, lose my mind. Barely a word was spoken on the way home. The only sound was me cracking, breaking down into the deepest, most painful sobs of my life.

"Why can't I just dance? I just want to dance! Why does everything have to be @*%$ taken away from me?!"

I was the very definition of insane.

"Why do I have to deal with so much *#$@?! I shouldn't have to deal with all this @*$%! $#*&! Why can't I just be %$#@ normal?!"

Life was way too painful at that moment. I wanted to die. I would never, ever, have killed myself during my journey, but there were countless times when I wished, and wanted, something else to. Sometimes, I wanted my heart to simply stop, and for all the physical and emotional pain to go away. Sometimes, I hoped for a relapse . . . a permanent relapse.

On the day before Good Friday, Mom researched the Maudsley approach. Heidi had introduced us to this form of treatment at our previous meeting, and by this time, Mom and I were open and willing to try anything.

Good Friday was pure hell, and Mom began to use this new approach. I sprawled on the floor by my bed, unable to think, hear, or see anything through my sobs. I had lost it so many times before, but it was suddenly so terrifying and real. Not an actual person, I only felt like a pile of broken pieces of who I once was. Every moment was excruciatingly painful, and each one only further chewed at my very spirit, like maggots in garbage.

Yelling and screaming, I blurted random things. It was as if I was a broken tape player, fast-forwarding, repeating, and jumping back and forth so it didn't make sense. Each thought, emotion, and feeling burned and stung, contributing even more to my loss of sanity. I have pondered so long, and so hard, how to describe what it felt like, lying in a heap that day, but my mind will not reach into the dark depths and resurface with words demonic enough.

Mom sat next to me, helplessly watching her only daughter crumble to pieces. It hurt me to look at her . . . I hated myself for what I was doing to her. Even though I could not help it, I blamed myself for *my* pain causing *her* pain. It was too much for me. I wanted to be in pain alone. I almost wanted her to just let go of my hand, walk out, and go on living a happy, normal life, leaving me there to eventually die.

The thought of further corrupting her life sliced at my heart like a carving knife. Although I couldn't ever summon enough gratitude to thank her for staying with me, I wondered how and why someone would do such a thing—try to save me. Thinking I would spend the rest of my short life a psychotic, pained, disturbed, and dysfunctional member of society, I didn't know what to think as I looked into my mom's eyes. She was not going to leave me . . . ever. She was never going to give up on me. She told me, then, that she didn't care what she had to do . . . she was going to help me get better. Beginning to get tough with me, this is what she said.

"I don't care. I don't care if we have to sell the house and eat our way across the world. We're going to get you better! And I'm going to get tough, but I want you to know that it's not *you* who I'm going to get tough with, it's Mr. Stupid! That freakin' *liar. I'm going in after him! I'm doing it because I love you. He can no longer live in you . . . I won't let him!"*

Those words.
"I won't let him. I won't let him."

Wow. Suddenly, a new feeling came over me, swept past me, nearly knocking me over. She wouldn't let him. *She wouldn't let him.*

It was right at that instant that I realized I was not alone and didn't have to fight all by myself. Mom was going to battle him. Just then, that fear of not listening to the evil voice was taken away. The trust I had in Mom crushed it all. She knew what was best for me . . . she was going to take care of me. I'll never, ever, forget what she did. Drawing an imaginary line in my fading carpet, she explained the truth.

"Now, on this side is Mr. Stupid. He is lies, untruths, hatred, and evil," she told me, pointing to one side of the line.

"And over here," she switched sides and pointed, "is the truth. It is love, and everyone who loves you . . . God, me, Nicholas, Dean, Dad, Gramma and Poppy, everyone at dance . . ."

I stared at where she pointed.

"Now, who are you going to trust . . . some guy who is full of $#%, or the people who love you?"

Tears flowed from my eyes and all the way down my cheeks before free-falling off. What was I doing? What was I doing to the people who love me? I was being selfish. I was taking myself away from them, while they stood helpless. I then knew that if I could not muster up the strength to heal myself for me, I had to do it for the ones I love. I could no longer unintentionally hurt my loved ones by hurting myself.

Honestly, I didn't care about myself or choose to do it for me. I pretty much hated myself, but apparently, there were people who needed me, wanted me, and loved me. I couldn't disappoint them; I couldn't break their hearts.

Then came a moment that will forever remain clear in my mind. Mom told me to look in her eyes.

After my many awkward, hesitant attempts, she commanded, "Look in my eyes!"

I did. She just stared, and I stared back. I felt I couldn't breathe. Her eyes were serious and focused, yet there was love in them . . . love so intense, I felt it deep within my soul. I felt vulnerable as I gazed deep into her eyes, and it was almost as if, rather than looking into each other's eyes, we were looking at each other's spirits.

The only words which rang in my heart were, "Thank you . . . thank you."

Before writing this, I asked Mom to describe what happened on this day. She paused before concluding with the only thing she could relate it to.

"An exorcism of Mr. Stupid—the devil himself."

And so, it seemed, on that same day that Jesus had been crucified and died on the cross, the dark, suffering part of me also died.

"Food is an important part of a balanced diet." —Josh Billings

TWENTY-FIVE

WITH EASTER came the rebirth, the rise of goodness, hope, and love. Of course, I still cried, broke down, and struggled, but I had completely thrown myself into battle toward health, happiness, and recovery. From this point on, life rolled down its runway and began to take off.

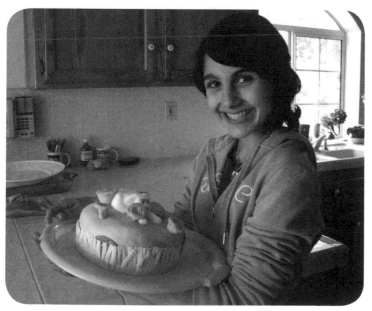

Proud of my Easter cake.

God placed many events in my life that showed me I was meant to live and also that served as an almost "reward" for the hard work I put toward recovery. I received a school district writing award for a poem I wrote in English class about *The Odyssey*, I danced in my school's Dance Company's show, and I accepted academic year-end awards for the freshman class in Health, Algebra II, and Top Ten GPA at Nipomo High School's Titan Award Night.

In May, I hit my one-year anniversary of the end of my treatment. The girl who had wanted to die just a month before now celebrated life with overwhelming gratitude. I returned to the Annual Rancho Oso Family Fun Day, only this time, with a full head of hair.

My fifteenth birthday came and went, tricking my mind into thinking I was still fourteen. But what I remember most about that May was the Teddy Bear Cancer Foundation's Grizzly Bear Breakfast. The Grizzly Bears are a group of businesspeople who support Teddy Bear. Nikki and Marni asked me to speak, so Mom and I arrived at Moby Dick's Restaurant in Santa Barbara on a clear, crisp May morning.

The salty sea air refreshed me as I took a deep breath, holding a brand-new speech tightly in my hands. I had decided to lay it all on the line, not hold back, and share with these people exactly what it is I went through, and how the Teddy Bear Cancer Foundation helped me. Stepping up to a high wooden podium, I asked God to help me keep it together. After pausing for a moment, I began:

> "We have diagnosable tissue," my Dr. Dan told us, referring to my second biopsy. The first one proved to be unsuccessful. This was December 18, 2007, the day we finally discovered that the huge mass in my chest was Hodgkin lymphoma. Nine days later, I was violently thrown into the world of a cancer patient. I began my first of four rounds of chemotherapy, each consisting of three days in the hospital and a fourth day at the clinic. I was swept off my feet over and over, yet I still clawed my way to the surface, with the support of my friends and family. Part of this family is the Teddy Bear Cancer Foundation, who, with each selfless, kindhearted act, wedged

themselves deeper into my heart and soul. They have assisted my family in countless ways, but one fairly recent event truly brings tears to my eyes.

I had completed my chemo, and three long weeks of daily radiation, on May 8, 2008. Although excited to be finished with treatment, I faced a battle just as difficult . . . recovery. Struggling with late effects, I became extremely depressed. I was so confused that one must recover from what actually cured them . . . it didn't make sense. My mind was in a gray zone, hovering between sick one day and semi-well the next.

As time pushed on, I began to feel worse and worse, and my depression became so bad that not even I, let alone my family, recognized me. I used to be funny and joyful, not the girl curled in a ball on the floor crying, or the girl who stood for minutes and minutes at a time—her head against the living room wall. We started to investigate my symptoms and found out that everything I was feeling corresponded to a list of side effects from one of my medications. I stopped taking it immediately, and some of my symptoms subsided.

However, during the four or so months that I suffered, I began to develop a serious eating disorder. Each time food dropped into my stomach, I would endure intense pain, and other terrible symptoms, from my medication. Therefore, I learned to hate anything edible and slowly began wasting away because of the horrible associations I had ingrained in my mind. Also, the combination of the trauma of treatment and complete lack of control in my life contributed greatly.

As months rolled past, it became a serious situation. Only seventy-nine pounds at my lowest point, I was barely eating what many consider a snack in a day. The emotional pain was excruciating, like nothing I had ever experienced. The zest for life that used to burn so brightly inside of me was blown out, with only ashes remaining. I felt like I could not take any more suffering and each morning awoke intimidated and scared about what struggles the day would bring. My mind, so scarred from all that it had been through, saw an orange as a meal, skinny as fat, and anything enjoyable as bad for me.

I had two voices in my head: the part of me that wanted to get well and to heal, and the part that wanted to see me suffer. I was so confused. I wholeheartedly wanted to become healthy and strong once again, but an invisible, evil, controlling something held me back. It was as if I had gotten so used to being in pain, I felt that if I was not, then I wasn't trying hard enough. I became a slave to my very own mind, and deep down, I was terrified and screaming for help. But when my mouth came open, no words came out, for there were truly no earthly words that could possibly explain what was happening to me.

In October 2008, I spoke at the Teddy Bear Cancer Foundation luncheon, and only three days later, I told my mom I needed help. I was so scared; I didn't know how to do it myself. Mom researched immediately, finding an eating disorder specialist and registered dietician in our area. The therapist seemed perfect, and I had a speck of hope. But there was a problem. The therapist did not accept our insurance, and the appointments were very expensive. Teddy Bear heard of my situation, and I'll never forget what my mom told me.

"The Teddy Bears are going to pay for it."

I cried so hard—huge, grateful, thankful tears. It meant more than the entire universe to me. It was hope. It was healing. It was my future. Having come such a long way since then, I am only more in love with these amazing people. Their hearts reached right in and grabbed mine. That was my only chance to get well, and without them, I shudder to think of where I would be now. They have indirectly given me back my spirit, my love, my joy, and my life. I am eternally grateful. I have never spoken of my eating disorder publicly before, but I chose to do so today to be a visual representation of a life touched by their warm, comforting, fuzzy paws.

Looking up from my speech, I saw rows of crying businesspeople through the blur of my own tears. I know the whole thing was probably awkward for them, as it was for me, but I wanted the truth to be known. Cancer kids need just as much help after treatment as during. We're like giant walking wounds, with each touch stinging and painful. Only time can make the wound scab over and begin to heal. But during that vulnerable time, we need a Band-aid. Teddy Bear was my Band-aid.

A standing ovation brought back memories of the October luncheon . . . there was a beautiful feeling in the room. I had never seen so many grown men crying like that, especially all at once. So many thanks and comments followed, and I remember one in particular, from a very loving man.

"You just make it so easy to write the check!" he admitted, with pools of moisture still lingering in his eyes.

That one sentence meant the world to me. To be able to help those other cancer kids and families was incredible. I began to realize, then, that it was only me who could do what I did. God gave me my story and journey so that I can know exactly what those kids go through, and I can help them through others. If I reached in and gracefully grabbed a businessman's heart, made him cry, and practically wrote the check for him, it was God's work. God was using the combination of my story, and my ability to share my story, as a tool to help all of His cancer kids.

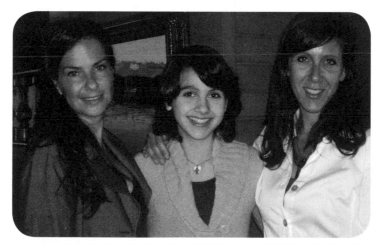

A moment of gratitude with Marni and Nikki at the 2009 Grizzly Breakfast.

It all made sense to me. I've been told people still talk about my speech that day and how I "made all the businessmen cry." It makes me laugh and recall what one man who had heard me speak the previous October had to say.

"When I saw you walk in," he told me, "I thought, 'Oh no! She's gonna make me cry again!'"

Ha, ha, ha . . . life is funny.

⌒

June came, and with it came the end of school and Dean's graduation. I couldn't believe it as I watched him, only a distant, red dot in a cap and gown, walking across the stage. Where had all the time gone? I still remembered when he was barely a junior, when I started feeling ill. Once again, time had slipped away from me like a wet bar of soap. Pyyyooo! Gone.

Also that month was the San Luis Obispo Civic Ballet audition. I had worked my buns off for it, and I was ready to give it my all. I can still remember the night I arrived home after three hours of dance and became suddenly inspired to choreograph my very own variation for the audition. It was nearly 11:00 at night when I collapsed, exhausted, on the living room floor. It was done. Finished. I loved it.

⌒

My mom and I traveled to Irvine to meet up with Priscilla and her daughter, Tanya. Our incredible friends from Washington have supported me every step of the way. Priscilla, unfortunately, was in extremely poor health, and when I was asked whether or not I wanted to go, I did not even take a single second to think about it. I had to go. I had not seen her in nearly five years, and I had to go thank her.

I'll tell you, just to put my arms around her, look into her bright hazel eyes, and show her my gratitude was unbelievable. Amazing. Funny thing, too, I suddenly had a new sense of compassion for her. Always having felt sorry that she had to go through all that she went through, I now had a different feeling toward her. It was as if I could not only see her pain, but feel it as well. I know what it is like to be that sick.

Auntie Priscilla, you are incredible, and I love you so, so much. You have done so much for me, and I am at a loss for words to express my gratitude. You are so strong, and you have a heart of pure gold.

Going to see her helped me to remember to cherish every step, every breath, and every improvement in my recovery. I was reminded that, although life is so, so tough, and I've been through the wringer, I still have so much to be grateful for.

⁀

Staring out at the snowy Rocky Mountains in the distance, I felt almost a tickle in my spirit. Yes, I was in Colorado, standing out on my hotel room balcony. As I took in the panoramic view, I thought back to when Robyn had asked me if I wanted to go with the Sunshine Kids. The Sunshine Kids take cancer kids various places and give them the time of their lives. That is exactly what I had—the time of my life.

With thirteen other kids—three from Sacramento, four from Texas, four from Kentucky, and three others from my Santa Barbara group—we spent six days in Steamboat Springs, Colorado. It was incredibly beautiful there, with huge, green fields and puffy, cotton-ball afternoon clouds. So many memories were made during those short six days, and the people I met were remarkable. One of these amazing people was my roommate, Mary, whose friendship I would not exchange for anything in the whole world.

I was very thankful I was healthy enough to go, and never would I have guessed, as I rolled into the OR, or got hooked up to another bag of chemo, that I would be standing in Colorado a year later because of it. Cancer has so many "bads," but this trip for me was yet another confirmation that there are "goods" as well.

It was a once-in-a-lifetime adventure. We rode a gondola up to over nine thousand feet and stared out at what seemed like the entire world. We went rafting on the Elk River. I can still feel the invigorating rush of the glacial water soaking me. We had VIP seats at the Steamboat Rodeo, and I got a kick out of the Colorado cowboys—they were straight out of a movie. One day our group traveled to Steamboat Lake, paddling kayaks and canoes before eating lunch on pontoon boats in the middle of the huge lake. I'll always remember the gorgeous, majestic 360-degree view of the snow-kissed mountains and approaching storm clouds in the distance.

Speaking of storms, one of my greatest memories of the trip was riding my horse, Ladybug, at Saddleback Ranch while rain poured down upon us. It was one of those moments where I stopped, and time seemed to stop as well. I looked around and tried to grasp where I was and what was happening. Bright green fields and hills surrounded us for miles, and I could see the slanted angle of the sheets of rain that were drenching us.

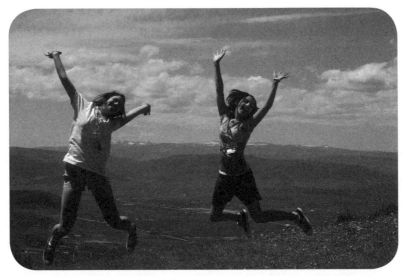

Mary and I on top of the world in Steamboat Springs, Colorado.

God's world was so big, beautiful, and powerful right then, and I felt like a mere speck on His massive globe. Somehow, although I felt tiny on the inside, I felt big. A harmonious feeling in my spirit made me feel as if I was meant to be in that exact spot, at that very second.

After leaving Colorado, I flew to Los Angeles and hopped on a little tin can to fly north to Santa Barbara. That baby rattled and shook like a rusty shopping cart—it scared the bejeebies out of me. Reunited with Mom, I retold all of my experiences to her as we drove north and arrived at the Relay for Life Luminaria Ceremony.

It was déjà vu as I walked around the track holding Mom's hand.

"In memory. In memory. In memory."

Wow, it hit me just as hard as it had the year before. Then, I came upon a different-looking luminary bag.

"Cancer Survivor," it read.

My heart soared.

"Melinda Marchiano."

Gramma and Poppy had lovingly created an "In Honor of" bag for me.

All the feelings came back to me: the guilt, the pride, the hope, the gratitude, the loss—it all formed a strange barnacle on my heart. I prayed to God, at that moment, that I would be standing in that same place, looking at a similar bag, years into the future.

Hope for that dream came as I received the results from my one-year check-up. Cancer free. Perfect. Beautiful. Every grain of thankfulness inside of me united to make a private beach of gratitude.

Another blessing came on June 1, 2009. I sat on that tan, leather couch in Heidi's office, gazing at the same dreaded objects . . . I didn't like it there anymore. It all brought me back to a time I never wished to go back to; it was too pain-ful. Being there made me remember the many days I sat there sick, dying, and pretty much insane. I could feel it . . . it had all stayed and lingered in the room like a foul stench. But the blessing came when I heard these words brush past Heidi's lips.

"Well, I don't think I need to see you anymore."

At that instant, an exhausted sense of pride punched me. I had won another battle, slain another Goliath. Heidi called it my "graduation," and I watched as she shuffled around her desk before turning to face me. She held in her hand a small, green and purple rock in the shape of a heart. Placing it in my palm, she explained why she had chosen the rock. There were cracks visible on the inside, but on the outside, all of these cracks became part of a larger, smooth heart shape. This was me: with cracks and scars on the inside, but, somehow, all of those marks formed me as a whole.

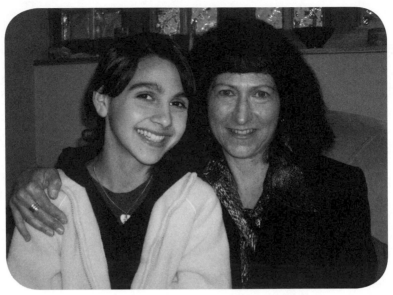

Me and Heidi, who helped heal my spirit.

"To get through the hardest journey we need take only one step at
a time, but we must keep on stepping." —Chinese Proverb

TWENTY-SIX

NOW, I CANNOT IMAGINE myself without all I have gained, and lost, through cancer. Most everyone who has cancer reacts differently to it. Some get mad that it ever happened, while some say it's the greatest gift they've ever gotten. I'm neither . . . I'm somewhere in between.

I have learned more about myself, others, the world, and life in two years than I will learn the rest of my days. But what it took to learn those things was the lowest, darkest, deepest, most painful time you could ever imagine. Was it worth it *then*? Heck no.

I didn't even know that God was trying to teach me something half the time . . . I processed and sorted it all out afterward. Still, I think back to a time in my journey and learn something that my oblivious, exhausted, or occupied mind did not grasp at the time. Yes, cancer is a roller coaster, and it seems that when you're not at the highest or the lowest point, you're in rapid transit either up or down.

I'm still waiting for my life to "even out," but frankly, I'm not sure it ever will. Cancer has changed me physically, spiritually, mentally, and emotionally. I compare myself to the life of a butterfly. I was a naive, little caterpillar, slipped into a chrysalis and then morphed into a beautiful butterfly. That butterfly may have a bum wing, or only one antennae, but it is still beautiful in my mind.

Cancer has changed my thinking and has given me a crystal-clear picture of life and all of its meanings. I see now, more than ever, how vital it is that we love and be kind to one another, for anything can happen at any moment. We must help one another through this difficult, yet incredible, life and be compassionate and understanding.

I've also been taught how little, tiny acts of kindness can make a huge impact on someone's life. Having been touched this way by so many along my road, it inspires me to do the same in others' lives. We never know what people are going through, or how much even the simplest smile can mean to them.

Everyone has their own unique challenges, and this brings me to another thing I've learned. It is the importance of love, laughter, and kindness during difficult times. It is easy to get wrapped up in our struggles and turn sour, but it is at this moment that positive energy needs to build and shine through. I cannot tell you how many times I laughed during my journey when, really, I shouldn't have. Sometimes, I didn't even know what I was laughing at. Maybe it was God's way of protecting me emotionally. I'm not sure.

And, did you know, not once throughout the entire two-year process did Mom and I fight, or even clash? Surrounding ourselves with loved ones and drawing closer to them, instead of isolating and distancing ourselves from them, makes the love between us grow. Mom and I have always been so, so close, and we managed to pull in even closer through it all.

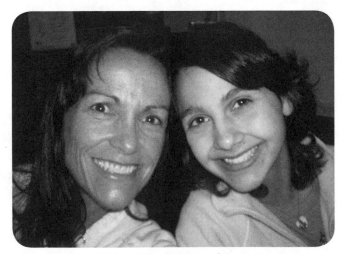

My best friend, twin, and mom.

Compassion, kindness, and understanding complete the magic potion of conquering tough times. I learned the difficult way, always having been extremely hard on myself. Finally, I realized that, as well as treating others with kindness, we need to be kind and compassionate toward ourselves. I would get so frustrated with myself, which only added stress and more frustration to my bucket of problems. Of course, the other extreme, self-pity, is no good either. It is a delicate balancing act between being our own worst enemy and sinking in the quicksand that is our very own empathy. And when we have that strength and foundation of love, humor, and compassion, we can accomplish just about anything.

When I was a little kid, I was scared of dying. Just the topic of death was very scary to me. This is another way I've been changed. I'm not afraid to die; actually, I think I'm looking forward to it. That thought in no way implies I'm suicidal, but I picture death now as more of a freedom—a release.

I know God knows the exact time, down to the second, when I will die, and I couldn't care less if it is in seventy years, twenty years, or two days . . . as long as it is God's time to take me to heaven. It is obvious that I want to live my life, and be here with my family, but I know that, when my time comes, it will be peaceful, angelic . . . spiritual.

I can only imagine being spared of all the pains of life, stripped away from my outer, human shell, until only my bare, naked spirit remains. I think some people are afraid to die because they're "not ready to go" and believe they have more life to live and more things to learn. Having learned so much myself, I feel that life is almost like going back to college after I already graduated. Now, of course, I can learn so much more . . . major in something else. And when I get *that* degree, I'll go back and major in something else. I want to learn everything about the world. So I guess I'm not afraid of dying because I feel as if I did already pass. I will look back on my life so far and be happy for what I've done and be fulfilled with what God has taught me. I will be satisfied. But that doesn't mean that every day, from here on out, isn't going to be lived to the fullest . . . just watch me.

You are probably thinking, "If she is okay with dying, where did she get the willpower to live?"

Three words: Those I Love.

They were my source of strength and what I remained strong for. I battled for my life, really, only so I could still be a part of their lives. Any moment I would wish to die was suddenly and completely extinguished by this thought:

"What about my family?"

They were my willpower and the glue that held me together. Several times I imagined those I know and love without me in their lives or them in mine. I remember the night I was rushed to the ER, as I fought to remain conscious.

"@*$%! I'm not gonna die! I'm not gonna @*$% die!" I screamed in my head.

As I held my brother's hand and stared into his dark brown eyes, I couldn't leave him. I didn't give a you-know-what about me . . . I couldn't leave *him* at that moment. I couldn't break his heart like that. So many times, I didn't care about myself and had to be reminded that I needed to, because people love me. I put myself in their shoes, watching someone they cared so deeply about wanting to give up on their life . . . it broke my heart. I had to win. I fought for what made me happy, and that was every single person in my life who I love.

Loved ones, and one other source of happiness, kept me going. I bet you know what that is—*dance*. Patricia Barker wrote in her letter to me that I would return to dance with a new energy, love, and passion. Ms. Barker, you were right. I find myself in class loving every turn, every *tendu*, every *developpé*, and even every stumble, tangle, or fall. *Grand allegro* is one of my favorites. There is that one instant, when I am at the peak of a huge leap, that I feel entirely weightless, with nothing but the feeling of pure gratitude and the air rushing past me. It is at these moments that I thank God I am alive . . . and dancing. It was all of those days when I arrived at class with a broken heart, and a sick, weak body, that my love for dance grew even greater.

This brings me to another subject . . . gratitude. As you can imagine, thankful-ness is within me, and radiating outward every instant. Every second of every day, I am grateful. Many minds cannot grasp what it truly means to be thankful for every waking moment. Only a handful of people emit this gratitude through their hearts and spirits, hoping dearly to teach those who do not know of the unfathomable preciousness of life.

Here are some things that I have become grateful for . . .

Taking a step
Opening my eyes and being able to see God's beautiful world
Taking a deep breath
Not even taking one single pill a day
Reading something and comprehending it
Going to a store and being able to fit into clothes
Making cookies and knowing I can have one
Seeing muscles form on my body again . . . everywhere
Not being afraid of how I will feel
Cracking a joke because I have the energy
Sitting upright, not having to lie down
Being warm-blooded again
Having hair
Being able to smile

There are so many more and I could, seriously, go on forever—from every-day things, to people in my life, to the technology and scientific advances that helped save me. To me, I am the most blessed person on this planet.

☙

Along with the things I gained also came loss. I still randomly find myself griev-ing over what I have lost. It is a painful grief, as though someone has died, or something tragic has happened. That person who died was the old me, and that tragedy was—everything I once knew was taken from me.

Two years of my life were snatched up, and I wonder to this day what would have happened if I didn't get cancer. What would my life be like? Strangely, I can't picture it, so I guess this is how I am supposed to be. But still, it does not stop me from missing the "old me" and my old life. Everything changed when I got sick, and it hasn't been, and will never be, the same. I went from a happy, normal thirteen-year-old, to someone with a life of worry, anxiety, and responsibility. To suddenly be exposed to so much at a tender age is frightening. I felt like I had lost all innocence. I had to grow up so fast—I had no choice. I remember feelings I had when I was a kid: incredible, carefree feelings deep down in my soul. How I long for one tiny speck of one of those moments. When I was little, the hardest decision I had to make was what stuffed animal I wanted to play with.

Suddenly, little Melinda was fighting for her life. And now, I have to be truthful, I am in many ways haunted by it. I am overwhelmed that the bad memories will always be with me. But, like the stone Heidi gave me, even the struggles and challenges I faced have shaped me into the person I am today. And although I so greatly miss the life I used to have, I must not live in the past, which brings me to yet another lesson I've learned.

The time is now. We all need to live in each second, without agonizing over the past or anxiously awaiting the future. It seems, so many times, that many of us have trouble with this concept . . . even me. It is easy to let time pass us by as we are unknowingly living in the past or waiting for that "perfect time" in the future. Really, "now" is all we will ever have, and so, we need to acknowledge and accept that. Right when I write this, it is "now," but as I complete this sentence, that "now" has suddenly been replaced with a new "now." We are not time travelers, and think about it . . . all of our memories were once a "now." It just shows us how important "now" is.

Of course, looking forward to things or evoking wonderful memories from times past is great, but I began to realize, lying in that hospital, that I didn't want to just "get through" my days. I wanted to live them and not throw away the precious days God gives to me. They are short . . . way too short.

⌒

Having battled an eating disorder, new light has been shed on what these disorders are, and what they do. I always thought it was only freakishly thin girls, starving themselves to look like their favorite model, who were victims. Now I know what it truly is. It is like an addiction in the sense that once one starts starving themselves, they cannot stop. It feels good . . . somehow it brings a sick sense of pleasure. People with eating disorders do not know that they are killing themselves, and not just physically . . . they are killing their spirits as well.

I'll never forget lying in bed at night, my heart beating what seemed like every ten seconds. I felt so faint, and I could have sworn my heart skipped beats. I know now, it could very well have stopped . . . quit. Having experienced some of the worst emotional moments imaginable, I realize how out of control one's thoughts can be. Many people believe that a person with an eating disorder wants to think what they think, but, personally, I found my thoughts to be uncontrollable. I didn't know why that stuff entered my mind. I didn't want to think like that . . . I just did.

It can be so scary when our minds become independent of us. One day I became so extremely frustrated I purposely hit my head on the wall. Afterward, I became nauseous . . . I think I gave myself a concussion. Two words can describe how I felt at that time in my life: miserable and terrified. At one point, I began to want to go to dance only to lose weight, but I love dance so much, I didn't want my relationship with it to be like that.

Eating disorders rip everything away from you. They control you, and your life, to such an extent it *is* your life. They are the very devil himself—so evil that words cannot be used to describe them. Only courage, determination, faith, and intense fighting will finally show someone what life really is, and how beautiful it is. I received my life back, and it is truly impossible to explain how it feels to be free, released from the chains of my eating disorder.

☙

Faith played a very strong role in my battle. I don't believe that I beat cancer but that God beat it, and I had to remain strong for Him. Through the whole, entire thing, I have never felt so close to—and so far away from—God. There were times when I could practically feel His gentle, comforting touch, and other times where I had to keep pushing to believe that He was still there. But whenever I questioned my faith in God, He always showed me, in some small way, that I was in His loving hands. On so many occasions, I would yell out to God for help or for strength, and I didn't even realize He was right next to me.

You know, when you're calling out to someone and they're like, "Whoa, whoa, I'm just right here!"

That's what God said to me throughout my fight. I know that I would not be here if not for His unfathomable grace. During my eating disorder, He was one of my only comforts, and so many times I begged for His gentle, loving touch to keep me sane. And that verse . . . that Bible verse filled me.

"Do not be anxious about anything, but in everything, by prayer and petition, with thanksgiving, present your requests to God. And the peace of God, which transcends all understanding, will guard your hearts, and your minds, in Christ Jesus."
—Holy Bible, New International Version, Philippians 4:6

Wow. Think about it. Anything. *Anything.* This one single verse brought me through so many trying times, I've lost count. My gratitude toward God is beyond gratitude. I have come so much closer to Him than I have ever been—a priceless gift cancer gave to me. I will do anything to show Him how much I love Him and how grateful I am for all He has done for me. Since my illness began, not a single time at church has gone by that I haven't balled my eyes out. God is a part of me, and always will be. He saved me for a reason, and kept me on this Earth to do something—He has a plan for my life. Although I do not, or may never, know why or what I was chosen to live for, I will always do one thing . . . spread His love and His grace everywhere I go.

And so, here I am, a "normal," healthy, fifteen-year-old girl, with an incredible story behind her two brown eyes. I've had forty-eight doses and sixteen days of chemo, well over fifty tests, a trip to the ER, two doses of morphine, three drug reactions, forty-one shots, over 150 needle pokes, fourteen days of radiation, an eating disorder, a mass the size of a softball, a PICC line, a port, two biopsies, a bone marrow aspiration, total hair loss, nine months of intense therapy, and so many doctor's appointments that I lost count a year ago.

Now, I have written a book. My dance bag is slung over my shoulder, right this instant, and I am getting ready to go dance my soul out for two straight hours . . . I can't think of a better way to celebrate. My heart is filled with a nearly indescribable feeling at this moment. It can only be described with one word . . . *grace*.

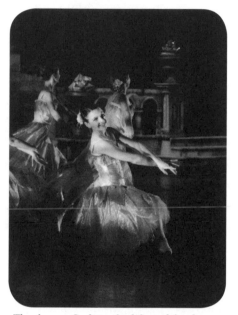

Thank you, God . . . for life and for dance.
Nutcracker 2009.
Photo by Julie Campbell.

"And He has said to me, 'My grace is sufficient for you, for power is perfected in weakness.' Most gladly, therefore, I will rather boast about my weakness, so that the power of Christ may dwell in me."
—New American Standard Bible, II Corinthians 12:9

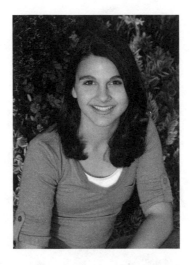

Melinda Marchiano lives in the rolling, oak-studded hills of the Central Coast of California. Homeschooled through the eighth grade, she enjoyed from a young age the freedom to write and create. Now in high school, she is academically at the top of her class. Melinda dances six days a week and performs with the Civic Ballet of San Luis Obispo and with San Luis Jazz. A childhood cancer survivor, she gives thanks for her life by speaking and fundraising for such organizations as the Teddy Bear Cancer Foundation, the Children's Miracle Network, and the American Cancer Society's Relay for Life.